DRUGS IN CURRENT USE 1958

drugs

IN CURRENT USE

Edited by

WALTER MODELL, M.D., F.A.C.P.

*Associate Professor, Clinical Pharmacology, Cornell University
Medical College*

SPRINGER SCIENCE+BUSINESS MEDIA, LLC 1958

ISBN 978-3-662-39273-7   ISBN 978-3-662-40303-7 (eBook)

DOI 10.1007/978-3-662-40303-7

Library of Congress Catalog Card Number: 55-1210

Price: $2.00

Quantity prices: 4 through 9 copies, $1.90 each

10 or more copies, $1.80 each

To receive your DRUGS IN CURRENT USE 1959
upon its publication in January 1959,
mail this coupon not later than December 1st, 1958.

Please send _____copies DRUGS IN CURRENT USE 1959, Modell $2.00*

Check (Money order) for $_____enclosed — post free
(add 3% tax in New York City)

Name ....

Address ....

....BB

* The $2.00 price and quantity prices in effect for all orders mailed before December 1st,
even if the 1959 edition should have a higher list price.

PREFACE

This is an annually revised alphabetical listing of drugs; well-established drugs, new ones still on trial, old ones of questionable or purely traditional value but still likely to be encountered; and, in addition, some drugs seen only as the cause of poisoning and some that are obviously doomed but which, for sentimental reasons, we are reluctant to discard. Inclusion of a drug in this list is not to be taken as a recommendation of utility but merely as a statement of the fact that it is being used. The number of new drugs appearing on the scene is great and, to keep up-to-date, annual revision has been found to be essential.

Our purpose is to provide a concise statement of the principal pharmacologic characteristics of drugs in current use; of their major uses; their physical properties; absorption; actions, both therapeutic and toxic; mode of administration; preparations; dosage; specific antidotes against poisoning when these are available— a capsule-account of the data essential to the sensible exploitation and safe handling of a drug. In some cases special warnings are noted which draw attention not only to dangerous reactions, contraindications, and questionable utility, but also to instability, special requirements for storage and prevention of deterioration, and to time limits before significant loss in potency or change in pharmacologic properties. In order to accomplish this in a compact form, the writing is terse; sentences are often incomplete. Very brief statements follow less commonly used or relatively untested drugs. When the properties of one drug are identical or very similar to those of another, the reader may be referred to the latter. In order to keep the book at its present convenient size and still deal with the large number of new drugs, reference is often made to remarks on old and well-established drugs in cases where they apply to new congeners.

Short essays on pharmacologic groups of drugs are also included in the alphabetic listing. These essays deal with problems of use, and actions and dangers characteristic of drugs as a group. The information here is often more detailed than that given for the individual drugs which may exhibit only minor variations from the properties of the group as a whole. A list of some of the available drugs in the group follows each essay which may also be used in conjunction with the statements on individual drugs. Some therapeutic groups of drugs in common use are also listed.

Usually only the drug principle is indicated; separate listings are rarely made of salts of the same basic drug. This is done to save space and to avoid useless repetition since the actions of drugs attach to their principle, and their salts usually differ only in physical properties, such as solubility or taste. For example, only the alkaloidal form of morphine is listed and there is no separate listing for the more commonly used soluble salt, the sulfate. Where practical differences do exist, the different forms are listed and described under the heading of the principle rather than separately.

In a compact book such as this, it is not possible to list all medicaments on the American market; there are too many, and many are merely minor variations on well-established themes. Inclusion in New and Nonofficial Drugs of the American Medical Association weighed heavily in deciding to include a proprietary preparation in this book.

Drugs are described under official names wherever these have been established. Because of widespread usage, proprietary names and synonyms could not be ignored in a realistic presentation; the more common ones are usually included, but their listing is by no means complete. In making such selections, many arbitrary decisions had to be made, and it was usually on the basis of the Editor's judgment and personal experience that one proprietary name for a drug was omitted and another included. Proprietary names are followed by the symbol®.

Only a few of the vast number of mixtures on the market are included. Immunologic agents such as the antigens, allergenic extracts, vaccines, toxins, toxoids, antitoxins, etc. are not included. Only a few representative solvents, vehicles, colors, flavors, emulsifying agents, and other pharmaceutic materials without significant pharmacologic action used in making up medicaments are included.

Dosage is usually indicated but it must be emphasized that a single value such as is usually given here can hardly apply to all patients. This is only the common dose given, but the range of useful dosage is far broader.

Many sources were used in compiling this list: the current as well as older editions of the United States Pharmacopeia (Mack Publishing Co.), National Formulary (American Pharmaceutic Association), Useful Drugs (Lippincott), the reports on New and Nonofficial Drugs as they currently appear in the Journal of the American Medical Association in the Reports of the Council on Drugs, and 'Modern Drug Encyclopedia (Drug Publications). From time to time, comments obviously based on personal opinion are to be found; these may be attributed to the Editor.

December 10th, 1957   *Walter Modell, M.D.*
New York

Rounded Dosage Equivalents for Metric and Apothecary Systems

Weights

Apothecary	Metric		
gr. $^1/_{200}$	0.0003 Gm.	or	0.3 mg.
gr. $^1/_{100}$	0.0006 Gm.	or	0.6 mg.
gr. $^1/_{60}$	0.001 Gm.	or	1.0 mg.
gr. $^1/_{50}$	0.0012 Gm.	or	1.2 mg.
gr. $^1/_{30}$	0.002 Gm.	or	2.0 mg.
gr. $^1/_{12}$	0.005 Gm.	or	5.0 mg.
gr. $^1/_8$	0.008 Gm.	or	8.0 mg.
gr. $^1/_4$	0.015 Gm.	or	15.0 mg.
gr. ss	0.03 Gm.	or	30.0 mg.
gr. i	0.06 Gm.	or	60.0 mg.
gr. iss	0.1 Gm.	or	100.0 mg.
gr. ii	0.12 Gm.		
gr. iii	0.2 Gm.		
gr. v	0.3 Gm.		
gr. viiss	0.5 Gm.		
gr. x	0.6 Gm.		
gr. xv	1.0 Gm.		
gr. xxx	2.0 Gm.		

Liquid

Apothecary	Metric
♏ i	0.06 cc.
♏ ii	0.12 cc.
♏ iii	0.2 cc.
♏ v	0.3 cc.
♏ viiss	0.5 cc.
♏ x	0.6 cc.
♏ xv	1.0 cc.
♏ xxx	2.0 cc.
ʒ i	4.0 cc.
ʒ ii	8.0 cc.
℥ ss	15.0 cc.
℥ i	30.0 cc.
℥ ii	60.0 cc.
℥ iv	120.0 cc.
℥ vii	180.0 cc.
℥ viii	250.0 cc.
quart	1000.0 cc.

A

ACACIA—Gum Arabic
Emulsifying agent. A gum, which occurs in tears, fragments or powder. Slowly soluble in water.
Actions and Uses: Used sometimes as a demulcent, but chiefly as an emulsant.

ACENOCOUMARIN—Sintron®
Anticoagulant. One of the coumarin derivatives, which see, said to have a curve of action between that of Dicumarol and Tromexan. Final evaluation requires considerably more experience.

ACETANILID
Analgesic and antipyretic. White powder, slightly soluble in water.
Absorption: Well absorbed from G. I. tract.
Actions and Uses: Although it has antipyretic actions and will reduce temperature, it is mainly used as an analgesic, often in headache remedies and similar mixtures. It relieves many common aches and pains, headaches, neuralgias, arthralgias, dysmenorrhea, myalgias. Effects are well developed within half an hour after oral dose. It is eliminated in a conjugated form in the urine.
Warnings: Its continued use may lead to the development of methemoglobinemia.
Administration: Oral.
Preparations: Tablet and powder. Compound acetanilid powder is a mixture of acetanilid, caffeine and sodium bicarbonate.
Dose: 0.2 Gm.

ACETARSONE—Stovarsol®
Antiprotozoal. White or yellowish powder, slightly soluble in water. Arsenical.
Actions and Uses: Used to destroy parasites in amebiasis and trichomonas vaginalis.
Warnings: In common with other arsenicals, may damage kidneys or liver.
Administration: Oral, vaginal insufflation.
Preparations: Tablet, 50, 100, 250 mg.

Powder, contains kaolin, sodium bicarbonate and acetarsone.
Dose: Oral, 0.25 Gm. 2 or 3 times a day, for 7 days. Vaginal insufflation, powder containing about 0.5 Gm. acetarsone in 4 Gm.
Antidote: Dimercaprol.

ACETAZOLEAMIDE—Diamox®
Diuretic. White powder, soluble in water.
Absorption: prompt and complete from the G.I. tract. Also the sodium salt.
Actions and Uses: Diuretic action is usually prompt. Useful in all cases in which diuretics are indicated. Used also in the treatment of glaucoma where a localized action may reduce intro-ocular pressure.
Effectiveness as anticonvulsant in epilepsy has been reported.
Warnings: Paresthesias of fingers and toes are common with use but these often disappear while the drug is continued. Agranulocytosis has been reported which is not surprising since drug is closely related to Sulfonamides, which see.
Administration: Oral, parenteral.
Preparations: Tablet, 250 mg. Vials, 500 mg.
Dose: 250 to 750 mg. daily in divided doses.

ACETIC ACID
Caustic and rubefacient. Clear, colorless solution containing about 36.5% acetic acid. It may be mixed with water, alcohol and glycerin. Has odor of vinegar and a sharp acid taste.
Actions and Uses: Used as a caustic and rubefacient and as antidote to alkali. Occasionally used to treat pediculosis.
Administration: Topical.
Preparations: Glacial Acetic Acid contains about 99.5% acetic acid. Diluted Acetic Acid contains about 6% acetic acid.

ACETOMEROCTOL—Merbak®
An organic mercurial antiseptic. See Mercury.
Antidote: Dimercaprol.

1

ACETONE
Solvent. Clear, colorless volatile fluid with a sweet taste. Miscible with water, alcohol, ether, chloroform. Used for cleansing.
Actions and Uses: Used as solvent and sometimes for cleansing instruments.
Warnings: Never used internally.

ACETOPHENETIDIN—Phenacetin
Antipyretic and analgesic. White crystalline powder with a bitter taste. Slightly soluble in water.
Absorption: Well absorbed from G. I. tract.
Actions and Uses: Effects are fully developed in about 30 minutes following oral administration. They may persist for about 3 hours. Although it has antipyretic properties, it is used mainly for its analgesic action, relieving many common and not very serious aches and pains, headaches, myalgias, neuralgias, arthralgias and dysmenorrhea.
Warnings: Its continued use may lead to methemoglobinemia. A common ingredient of the advertised pain remedies and cold cures.
Administration: Oral.
Preparations: Tablet and capsule.
Dose: 0.3 Gm. for adults.

ACETPYROGALL—Lenigallol®
Caustic. White powder insoluble in water.
Actions and Uses: Liberates pyrogallol slowly, producing painless corrosion.
Administration: Topical.
Preparations: Powder and ointment.
Dose: 5 to 10% concentration.

ACETRIZOATE—Thixokon®, Urokon®
Diagnostic. White powder, radio-opaque iodide, slightly soluble in water.
Actions and Uses: Excreted into urine and used in x-ray visualization of urinary tract and renal function tests. Also used for angiography and arteriography, including cerebral arteries.
Warnings: Same as for other iodine compounds.
Administration: Intravenous, retrograde.
Preparations: Ampules and vials, 30 to 50% concentration.
Dose: Varies with medication.

ACETYL - BETA - METHYLCHO - LINE, see Methacholine

ACETYLCARBROMAL—
Carbased®
Non-barbiturate, non-narcotic tranquilizer. Usefulness yet to be determined.

ACETYLDIGITOXIN—Acylanid®
Cardiac Stimulant. A recently introduced crystalline digitalis material derived from *Digitalis lanata.* Differs from digitoxin in more rapid curve of action and incomplete absorption; but in no real sense less toxic. Practical importance remains to be determined.

ACETYL-PARA-AMINOPHENOL
—Apamide®
Analgesic. One of the non-addictive analgesics, which see.

ACETYLPHENYLHYDRAZINE
Red cell depressant. Crystalline material, slightly soluble in water.
Absorption: Absorbed from G. I. tract.
Actions and Uses: Depresses formation of red blood cells, and is used for that purpose in treatment of polycythemia vera, a condition characterized by excessive formation of red blood cells.
Warnings: Depression of red cell formation may be excessive, and all blood formation may be inhibited. Slowly eliminated, tends to be cumulative.
Administration: Oral.
Preparations: Capsule.
Dose: Usually about 100 mg. daily for a week. After that, a maintenance dose is used, the size and frequency of which is determined for each case.

ACETYLSALICYLIC ACID
—Aspirin, Ecotrin®
Analgesic and antipyretic. Crystalline material which is slightly soluble in water.
Absorption: Well absorbed from G. I. tract.
Actions and Uses: Has entirely nonspecific antipyretic action, relieving all kinds of abnormally elevated temperatures, without effect on the cause of the temp-

erature. In small doses which do not produce behavior changes, it relieves many of the minor aches and pains, headaches, myalgias, arthralgias, neuralgias and dysmenorrhea. It affords good relief in the exquisite joint pains of rheumatic fever. In this condition, it is used in relatively large doses which simulates the symptoms of cinchonism. Its use in rheumatic fever often provides relief, not only from the pain, but also the joint swelling. It has no curative action, however. In part, at least, its effects may be due to an anti-inflammatory action. Effects of the drug develop fully in about 30 minutes after an oral dose. It is eliminated mainly in the form of salicylate in the urine, effects persisting for about 3 hours from a single dose.

Warnings: G. I. distress, due to irritation, is common after large doses. Also seen are symptoms of cinchonism: dizziness, ringing in the ears, impaired hearing, headache. Serious poisoning may resemble that of acidosis. Large doses may also depress the blood clotting mechanism and cause a tendency to bleeding.

Administration: Oral.

Preparations: Tablets, 0.3 Gm.

Dose: 0.3-0.6 Gm. In rheumatic fever, however, doses as high as 1 Gm. every 3 hours.

Antidote: Sodium bicarbonate to hasten elimination. Vitamin K or one of its synthetic substitutes for hypoprothrombinemia. Exchange transfusions have been effective in severe cases.

ACETYLSTROPHANTHIDIN

Cardiac stimulant. This is a new, partially synthetic, digitalis material whose action is even more rapid than that of ouabain. It can be used intravenously only. Its final position is not established.

ACETYL SULFISOXAZOLE—Gantrisin® Acetyl

The acetylated form of the drug is said to have all the antibacterial and physical properties of sulfisoxazole (Gantrisin®) but, in addition, to be especially free of intestinal irritant action and to be taste-less so that it is easily flavored for use in pediatric cases. Dosage of the same order as Sulfisoxazole, which see.

ACHROMYCIN V®, see Tetracycline, Phosphate Buffered

ACIBAN®, see Calcium Caseinate

ACIDIFIERS

Urinary: Ammonium chloride, Calcium chloride, Phosphoric acid, Sodium biphosphate.

ACIDORIDE®, see Glutamic Acid Hydrochloride

ACID SODIUM PHOSPHATE, see Sodium Biphosphate

ACIDULIN®, see Glutamic Acid Hydrochloride

ACONITE

Brown to orange powder derived from *Aconitum napellus.* Archaic drug.

ACRIFLAVINE

Antiseptic dye. Orange powder, freely soluble in water.

Actions and Uses: Used as an antiseptic dye and for its local action. It may be used to irrigate wounds, but more commonly it is used in treatment of gonorrheal urethritis. Since the advent of sulfa drugs and antibiotics, however, it is seldom used.

Administration: Topical.

Dose: Usually used in solution of from 1:1000 to 1:10,000 dilution.

ACRIZANE®, see Phenacridane

ACTH, see Corticotropin

ACTHAR®, see Corticotropin

ACTHAR GEL®, see Corticotropin

ACYLANID®, see Acetyldigitoxin

ADALIN®, see Carbromal

ADANON®, see Methadone

ADENOSINE-MONOPHOSPHATE —My-B-Den®

Nutritional. Recommended for a variety of conditions claimed to be due to poor tissue nutrition. Of questionable value.

ADIPHENINE—Trasentine®

Anticholinergic. White powder. The hydrochloride is soluble in water.

Actions and Uses: Much the same effect

on parasympathetic system as atropine and, hence, much the same uses and dangers. Said to have less mydriatic action than atropine.

Warnings: May produce mydriasis in sensitive patients.

Administration: Oral, rectal, intramuscular.

Preparations: Tablet, 75 mg. Ampule, 50 mg. in 1.5 cc. Suppository, 100 mg.

Dose: 75—150 mg.

ADRENAL CORTEX EXTRACT

Hormone. Hormone solution obtained from the adrenal glands of cattle.

Actions and Uses: May be used to replace missing cortical substances in Addison's disease or in any situation of cortical insufficiency.

Warnings: Toxic effects are rare in situations requiring cortical extracts. Overdosage may, theoretically, produce retention of sodium and symptoms akin to those of the edema of heart failure.

Administration: Subcutaneous, intravenous.

Preparations: Sterile injectable saline solution, free of fat and the epinephrine of the adrenals, containing only the cortical steroids. Vial, 50 Units per cc.

Dose: Expressed in Dog Units (based on the amount necessary to maintain the life of adrenalectomized dogs). The drug is usually given together with large amounts of saline and desoxycorticosterone. In a crisis an intravenous injection of 1250 Units (25 cc. of solution), although as much as 5000 Units, may be required within a few hours in severe cases. Further dosage is determined by the response to the first.

ADRENALIN®, see Epinephrine

ADRENERGICS

Epinephrine, Amphetamine, Cyclopentamine, Dextroamphetamine, Ephedrine, Ethylnorepinephrine, Hydroxyamphetamine, Isometheptene, Isopropylarterenol, Levarterenol, Mephentermine, Methamphetamine, Metaraminol, Methoxyphenamine, Methylhexaneamine, Naphazoline, Phenmetrazine, Phenylephrine, Phenylpropanolamine, Tanphetamine, Propyl-

hexedrine, Tetrahydrozolidine, Tuaminoheptane.

ADRENOCORTICAL HORMONES

Corticosterone, Desoxycorticosterone. See also Anti-inflammatory hormones.

ADRENOCORTICOTROPIC HORMONE, see Corticotropin

ADRENOLYTICS

Azapetine, Ergotamine, Ergotoxine, Hexamethonium, Phenoxybenzamine, Phentolamine, Piperoxan, Tetraethylamonium, Tolazoline.

ADRENOSEM SALICYLATE®, see Carbazochrome Salicylate

AEROSOL® PENETRATION CREAM

Creamy white ointment, readily miscible with water and easily removed from the skin by washing.

Actions and Uses: Used as a base for dermatologic drugs, in which penetration through the skin is needed. The cream penetrates hair follicles and pores.

AEROSPORIN®, see Polymyxin B

AGAR

Cathartic. Mucilaginous substance extracted from seaweeds. White, odorless and tasteless.

Absorption: Not absorbed from G. I. tract and passes unaltered into feces.

Actions and Uses: It is hydrophilic and swells when treated with water, absorbing and retaining water as it passes through the intestinal tract. It thus adds to the bulk therein and stimulates peristaltic activity.

Administration: Oral.

Dose: 4-5 Gm.

ALBAMYCIN®, see Novobiocin

ALBUMIN—Human Serum Albumin

Serum component of human blood. Clear brownish viscous liquid.

Actions and Uses: Raises the serum albumin content of the blood in hypoproteinemia. In edema due to low blood proteins, this reduces the edema accumulations. It may also be used in the treatment of shock.

Administration: Intravenous.

Preparations: Sterile solution.
Dose: Usually given in doses of about 25 Gm. for the adult, approximately 1 cc. per pound of body weight at a rate of not more than 2 cc. per minute. Usually given together with saline or 5% glucose.

ALCOHOL—Ethyl Alcohol
Solvent, rubefacient, astringent and antiseptic. Colorless, clear fluid containing about 95 % of pure alcohol. Inflammable. Has characteristic odor and taste. Is miscible with water, ether, chloroform and acetone.
Absorption: Rapidly absorbed from G. I. tract.
Actions and Uses: Applied to the skin, alcohol cools by evaporation and has a hardening or astringent action. It is an antiseptic at the concentration of 70% by weight; at all other concentrations its antiseptic action is weak. As an antiseptic, it requires time for action; after application, therefore, alcohol should be allowed to dry on the skin. Taken internally, it is quickly absorbed producing symptoms of intoxication in moderate doses. With this action, it has a sedative effect on some, it stimulates appetite in others, causes excitement in others and depression in still others. It is often difficult to anticipate the dosage necessary to produce an effect or the precise effect which may be produced unless one has had previous experience with the patient. Alcohol is completely metabolized in the body, providing a caloric content of about 225 calories per ounce. For this reason, alcoholic beverages tend to be fattening. It is also an important fact that alcoholics do not eat much of other foods, and the symptoms of alcoholic nutritional deficiencies are, in part, due to this action of alcohol.
Warnings: In large overdosage, alcohol produces narcosis. It may, if the dosage is very large, even cause death. Sudden withdrawal in chronic alcoholics may be followed by severe symptoms.
Administration: Topical, oral, intravenous.
Preparations: Solution.

Dose: External, 70% by weight. Internal, approximately 50% (approximately the concentration in 100 proof distilled liquors), in doses of 1-2 ounces.

ALDARSONE®, see Phenarsone

ALEVAIRE®, see Superinone

ALFLORONE®, see Fludrocortisone

ALGLYN®, see Dihydroxyaluminum Aminoacetate

ALGYN®, see Silver Protein

ALIDASE®, see Hyaluronidase

ALKAGEL®, see Aluminum Hydroxide Gel

ALKALIZERS
Urinary: Potassium acetate, Potassiur bicarbonate, Potassium citrate, Sodiur bicarbonate.

ALLYLBARBITAL—Sandoptal®
One of the rapid acting barbiturates which see.

ALMOND OIL, BITTER
Flavor. Volatile oil obtained from the same sources as the sweet almond oil. It is to be differentiated from the sweet almond oil, being volatile, having a char acteristic odor and taste given it by the benzaldhyde which it contains.
Actions ana Uses: Used only as a flav oring agent in medicaments.
Warnings: Contains small amounts of the poisonous hydrocyanic acid.

ALMOND OIL, EXPRESSED —Sweet Almond Oil
Emollient. Oil obtained from the kernels of several varieties of almond and related fruits. Clear, straw-colored or almost colorless and odorless. It is miscible with ether, chloroform and benzene.
Actions and Uses: Used for its emollient action on the skin.
Warnings: Do not use if rancid.

ALOE—Aloes
Cathartic. Yellow or brown powder obtained from the dried juices of the leaves of several species of aloe.
Actions and Uses: Mild cathartic, acting mainly on the large intestine.

Warnings: Large doses may produce renal irritation.
Administration: Oral.
Preparations: Pill.
Dose: 0.25 Gm.

ALOES, see Aloe

ALOIN
Cathartic. Light yellow powder, having a slight odor but an intensely bitter taste. Soluble in water and alcohol.
Actions and Uses: Used as a mild cathartic.
Warnings: Large doses may produce renal irritation.
Administration: Oral.
Preparations: Pill.
Dose: 15 mg.

ALPHAPRODINE—Nisentil®
A synthetic narcotic recommended as an analgesic with claims of rapid action, reduced incidence of nausea, vomiting, respiratory depression as compared with morphine. See morphine.
Antidote: Nalorphine.

ALSEROXYLON—Rau-Tab®, Rauwiloid®
A purified extract of Rauwolfia. Available in 2 mg. tablets.
Dose: 2-4 mg., 3 times daily.

AL-U-CREME®, see Aluminum Hydroxide Gel

ALUDRINE®, see Isoproterenol
ALUM
Astringent and hemostatic. Colorless crystals, fragments or a white powder. Sweetish to taste.
Actions and Uses: Chemically, alum may be aluminum ammonium sulfate or aluminum potassium sulfate. Strongly astringent, used as a styptic and hemostatic. May be used as a gargle.
Warnings: Seldom given internally. Somewhat injurious to the teeth when used as a gargle.
Administration: Topical.

ALUMINUM ACETATE
Astringent.
Actions and Uses: Used mainly in Burow's solution as an astringent. Burow's

solution contains about 5% of the aluminum acetate.
Administration: Topical.
Dose: Burow's solution as such; 0.5% solution in mouth washes.

ALUMINUM CARBONATE—Basaljel®
Another form of aluminum gel used as an antacid, with actions similar to aluminum hydroxide gel, which see.

ALUMINUM HYDROXIDE GEL —Alkagel®, Amphogel®, Al-U-Creme®, Creamalin®
Antacid. White suspension, containing approximately 4% of aluminum hydroxide.
Absorption: Not absorbed from G. I. tract.
Actions and Uses: Used mainly in peptic ulcer and as an alkali for functional hyperchlorhydria. It relieves pain by neutralizing the gastric acid. It neutralizes approximately 20 volumes of gastric hydrochloric acid. It does not tend to cause "rebound acidity." It reduces the formation of certain types of kidney stones.
Warnings: Prolonged use may interfere seriously with calcium absorption. Impaction of the gel in intestinal tract may cause obstipation or obstruction.
Administration: Oral.
Preparations: Liquid gel. Tablet 0.6 Gm. of the aluminum hydroxide. Mixture, with about 12% magnesium trisilicate which gives a gelatinous consistency and a mildly laxative action.
Dose: 8 cc.

ALUMINUM PENICILLIN
A slowly absorbed form of Penicillin G. See Penicillin.

ALUMINUM PHOSPHATE GEL —Phosphalgel®
Antacid. White, viscous suspension.
Actions and Uses: These are much the same as with the aluminum hydroxide gel, except that it provides phosphate in conditions in which this may be deficient

ALURATE®, see Aprobarbital

ALZINOX®, see Dihydroxy Aluminum Aminoacetate

AMALANONE—Amethone®
Topical anesthetic. Recommended for urologic diagnostic procedures.

AMARANTH
Dye. Dark red-brown powder, soluble in water.
Actions and Uses: Used in coloring foods and medicaments.

AMBENONIUM—Mytelase®
Cholinergic. A new drug with much the same sort of action as Physostigmine, which see. Advantages not yet clarified. Suggested for myasthenia gravis. Dosage of the order of 5 to 25 mg. orally although considerably more may sometimes be necessary.

AMBODRYL®, see Bromodiphenhydramine

AMETHONE®, see Amalanone

AMETHOPTERIN, see Aminomethyl-pteroylglutamic Acid

AMIDOPYRINE, see Aminopyrine

AMIGEN®, see Amino Acid Preparations

AMINITROZOLE—Tritheon®
Antiseptic. New drug used principally for trichomonas infections in both male and female, especially noteworthy because it appears to be effective taken orally. Final position in the therapy of this infection remains to be established. Available in 100 mg. tablets. Dosage of the order of 1 tablet three times a day for 10 days.

AMINOACETIC ACID—Glycocoll, Glycine
Nutritional. Amino acid. The body has an enormous capacity for the synthesis of glycine.
Absorption: Completely absorbed in intestinal tract.
Actions and Uses: May serve as a food. It was once thought that this amino acid might be a special and rapid source of energy and this was the basis of a fad for its use. In addition it appears that in some cases of myasthenia gravis and progressive or pseudohypertrophic muscu-

lar dystrophy, it may beneficially effect creatine metabolism. It has been largely superseded in these conditions by the much more effective neostigmine. Exerts a buffering action and may be used as an antacid as such, but usually with calcium carbonate.
Administration: Oral.
Dose: 30 Gm.

AMINO ACID PREPARATIONS
Nutritionals. These are usually mixtures of amino acids prepared by the digestion, acid or enzymatic, of various proteins; plasma, casein, lactalbumin, beef blood, liver, yeast. They occur as powders, usually with a bad taste, but often artificially flavored. Usually readily soluble in water, forming amber solutions. Amigen®, Aminonat®, Aminosol®, Hyprotigen®, Parenamine®, Protolysate®, Travamin®.
Actions and Uses: All the accepted amino-acid preparations contain the so-called essential amino acids in physiologic proportions. These are the essential stepping stones in building proteins in the body. Normally the body builds its proteins out of the amino acids it derives from the ingested foods. In special conditions where this is not possible, the amino acids may be used as dietary supplements. They are useful in the treatment of severe protein deficiency. When given intravenously as the only source of protein, the protein they supply seems to be labile and does not remain long in the body.
Warnings: Serious reactions may follow rapid intravenous injection. Large oral doses may cause severe diarrhea.
Administration: Oral, intravenous.
Preparations: Powder, solution.
Dose: The amount is determined by the degree of protein supplementation necessary. 1 Gm. protein per Kg. of body weight per day is considered adequate for an adult.

AMINO—METHYL-PTEROYL-GLUTAMIC ACID—Amethopterin, Methotrexate®
Anticarcinogenic. New drug available in 2.5 mg. tablets.

AMINOMETRADINE—Mictine®

An oral diuretic apparently prematurely introduced, now withdrawn from market because of unsatisfactory results. Replaced by a derivative of amisometradine (Rolicton®).

AMINONAT®, see Amino Acid Preparations

AMINOPENTAMIDE—Centrine®

One of the long list of anticholinergic drugs, with much the same actions and dangers as atropine, which see.

AMINOPEPTODRATE—

Caminoids®

A digest of liver, beef muscle, gluten, soya, yeast, milk proteins used as dietary supplement.

AMINOPHYLLINE—Theophylline Ethylenediamine

Diuretic, antispasmodic, respiratory stimulant. White or yellowish powder with a bitter taste. Relatively soluble in water.
Absorption: Relatively rapidly absorbed from G. I. tract.
Actions and Uses: It is used to dilate the coronary arteries in coronary thrombosis and insufficiency. There are many who question its usefulness in these conditions. It is also used to relax the bronchial musculature in asthmatic attacks. It is an effective diuretic, acting on the kidney to increase the rate of urine formation; a feeble respiratory stimulant.
Warnings: Given intravenously too rapidly, it may produce circulatory collapse; given at a moderated rate, prickling of the fingers may be noted. Given by mouth in effective diuretic doses, gastro-intestinal distress is exceedingly common.
Administration: Oral, intramuscular, intravenous, rectal.
Preparations: Tablet, 0.2 Gm. Solution, preparation for intramuscular injection is far too concentrated to be given safely by the intravenous route. Suppository.
Dose: Parenteral, 0.25-0.5 Gm. Oral or rectal: 0.2-0.6 Gm.

AMINOPTERIN

Bone-marrow depressant (folic acid antagonist). Indicated in the treatment of acute leukemia in children.

AMINOPYRINE—Pyramidon®, Amidopyrine

Analgesic and antipyretic. White crystalline material made synthetically. Slightly soluble in water.
Absorption: Well and rapidly absorbed from G.I. tract.
Actions and Uses: A dependable analgesic and antipyretic of the same pharmacologic group as aspirin. It relieves many of the common aches and pains listed under acetylsalicylic acid.
Warnings: In hypersensitive individuals, this drug and closely related drugs may cause serious and even fatal leukopenia and agranulocytosis. This condition may develop suddenly and without warning in patients who have taken the drugs previously without ill effect. Since there are usually many other drugs which can be easily substituted for these drugs, indications for its use are rare. On the other hand, it is important to determine whether new drugs are chemically related to aminopyrine.
Administration: Oral.
Preparations: Tablet, 0.2, 0.3 Gm.
Dose: 0.2-0.6 Gm.

AMINOSALICYLIC ACID, see Para-Aminosalicylic Acid

AMINOSOL®, see Amino Acid Preparations

AMISOMETRADINE—Rolicton®

Diuretic. New drug, replacing aminometradine (Mictine®) which apparently was not satisfactory. Value remains to be established by long clinical trial.

AMMONIA

Stimulant. A highly irritant caustic vapor, which dissolves easily in water. It has a characteristic ammoniacal odor. Strongly alkaline.
Actions and Uses: In solution, it is used as a chemical reagent. In the form of the ammonia spirit, it is used for its fleeting

action as a respiratory and circulatory stimulant, usually in cases of fainting.
Warnings: The solutions and vapors are highly irritant.
Administration: Inhalation.
Preparations: Ammonia solution, diluted, 10% solution in water. Ammonia solution, strong, 28% solution in water. Aromatic ammonia spirit, mixture containing about 2% of free ammonia with alcohol and aromatic oils.
Dose: Inhalation of the vapors of the aromatic spirit.

AMMONIATED MERCURY—White Precipitate

Local antiseptic. White powder.
Actions and Uses: Used externally as an antiseptic in infections of the skin.
Warnings: Excessive use may be irritant and may cause a dermatitis.
Administration: Topical.
Preparations: Cream, ointment with wax, petrolatum and other greasy or non-greasy bases. Mixed with salicylic acid and other drugs in skin ointments.
Dose: The dose is, to a large extent, determined by the strength of the ointment used. It should not be applied too liberally.

AMMONIUM ACETATE

Diaphoretic. Colorless or white crystals, slightly soluble in water.
Actions and Uses: Diaphoretic and diuretic drug of doubtful value and infrequently used.
Warnings: Overdosage may lead to acidosis.
Administration: Oral.
Preparations: Solution: Contains about 7% ammonium acetate and small amounts of acetic acid.
Dose: 15 cc.

AMMONIUM CARBONATE

Liquefying expectorant. Hard white or translucent masses having a strong ammoniacal odor and taste. It deteriorates on standing, losing ammonia and becoming opaque.
Actions and Uses: It is a nauseant, liquefying expectorant. Sometimes used, be-

cause of the free ammonia it gives off, as a reflex stimulant in "smelling salts."
Warnings: Strong alkali and irritant.
Administration: Oral.
Preparations: Tablet, pure ammonium carbonate. Aromatic spirit of ammonia, contains about 2% of ammonia, alcohol and aromatic oils. Mixture, cough medicines and expectorants.
Dose: Ammonium carbonate, 0.3 Gm. Aromatic spirit, 2 cc.

AMMONIUM CHLORIDE

Diuretic, acidifier and expectorant. Colorless or white crystals, with a cool or salty taste. Soluble in water.
Absorption: Rapidly absorbed from G. I. tract.
Actions and Uses: It is an irritant and nauseant. In common with all nauseants, it encourages bronchial secretion, hence used as an expectorant. In the body, it is changed into urea and free hydrochloric acid. The hydrochloric acid liberates sodium from the tissues, thus acting as a diuretic and increasing the rate of urine flow, and at the same time also acidifying the urine. Often used in conjunction with other diuretics, whose action it may intensify.
Warnings: Gastro-intestinal irritant with nausea and vomiting. Acidosis may occur in cases with poor renal function.
Administration: Oral.
Preparations: Tablet, 0.5 Gm., enteric coated. Mixture, with cough medicines.
Dose: Diuresis, 3–9 Gm. daily. Expectorant, 0.3 Gm.

AMMONIUM COMPOUNDS

The hydroxide and carbonate of ammonia are strong alkalis, and little used in medicine except for the stimulant action of their vapors, which are irritant on inhalation.
The neutral ammonium salts, such as ammonium chloride, are used because they are nauseant and, as such, are effective expectorants; they are also acid-forming salts, tending to acidify the urine. They act as diuretics, enhance the action of some of the diuretics and are used in conjunction with urinary anti-

septics, such as methenamine and mandelic acid, which are effective only in highly acid urine.

There is the danger in using the acid-forming salts in patients with reduced renal function, that the kidney may be unable to excrete the acid formed, and, as a consequence, acidosis may develop.

AMMONIUM HYDROXIDE, see Ammonia

AMMONIUM MANDELATE
Urinary antiseptic.
Actions and Uses: This is a form of mandelate which tends to acidify the urine. See Mandelic Acid.
Warnings: Excessive dosage may cause renal irritation and gastro-intestinal upset.
Administration: Oral.
Preparations: Tablet, Sirup, for children.
Dose: About 12 Gm. daily for adults.

AMNESTROGEN®, see Estrogenic Substances, Conjugated

AMNIVIN®, see Visammin

AMOBARBITAL—Amytal®
Hypnotic. White crystalline powder, insoluble in water, usually the soluble sodium salt. Bitter taste.
Absorption: Rapidly absorbed from G. I. tract.
Actions and Uses: Short-acting hypnotic and sedative, similar to barbital and phenobarbital, but with effects which develop more rapidly and which are eliminated more rapidly. Used to control insomnia and anxiety, but also used as a preliminary to surgical anesthesia. See Barbiturates.
Warnings: Overdosage may lead to narcosis and death. Regular use may lead to habituation. Abrupt withdrawal may lead to convulsions.
Administration: Oral, intravenous, intramuscular.
Preparations: Tablet, 50, 100 mg. Capsule, 0.065, 0.2 Gm.—sodium salt, is usually identified by a blue-colored capsule. Elixir, contains alcohol, coloring matter and flavoring matter, with about 25 mg.

amytal per teaspoon. Ampule, 0.25 and 0.5 Gm., to be dissolved before injection, into a 2% solution.
Dose: 30 mg. to 0.5 Gm., depending upon therapeutic indication.
Antidote: Picrotoxin.

AMODIAQUIN—Camoquin®
Antimalarial. The hydrochloride.
Actions and Uses: Much the same as chloroquine, which see.

AMPHETAMINE—Benzedrine®, Raphetamine®
Adrenergic. White powder, with a bitter taste, usually sulfate or phosphate, soluble in water. Amphetamine is volatile and has a characteristic odor.
Absorption: Rapidly absorbed from G. I. tract.
Actions and Uses: Used largely for its cephalotropic actions, stimulating mildly depressed states, producing a sense of well being, depressing the appetite, hence used in obesity, as an adjunct in the treatment of alcoholism, as a stimulant in barbiturate poisoning and depression. Often used to counteract sleepiness, narcolepsy, mental fatigue, orthostatic hypotension.
Warnings: Tends to elevate blood pressure. Excessive use, even early in the day, may produce insomnia.
Administration: Oral.
Preparations: Tablet, 5-10 mg. of the sulfate. Elixir.
Dose: 5 mg. twice a day.
Antidote: Barbiturates.

AMPHOGEL®, see Aluminum Hydroxide Gel

AMPHOTERICIN
New antibiotic under investigation; not available on the commercial drug market at this time.

AMPROTROPINE—Syntropan®
Anticholinergic. White powder, soluble in water, bitter taste.
Actions and Uses: Acts like atropine to depress parasympathetic influences, but much less potent. Used for peptic ulcer and intestinal hypermotility.

Warnings: May cause mydriasis in sensitive patients.
Administration: Oral, subcutaneous, intramuscular.
Preparations: Powder. Tablet 100 mg.
Dose: 100–200 mg.

AMYLENE HYDRATE
The solvent for tribromoethanol (Avertin®) in anesthesia.

AMYL NITRITE
Vasodilator. Clear yellowish liquid with a characteristic fruity odor and a pungent taste. Volatile and inflammable.
Absorption: Almost instantaneously absorbed when inhaled, with immediate effects.
Actions and Uses: Dilates smooth muscle more especially that of the coronary arteries, which makes for its outstanding use to relieve the pain of angina pectoris (due to spasm of the coronary arteries). Also used as an emergency measure in the treatment of cyanide poisoning, to produce methemoglobinemia. Effects persist for a short time only.
Warnings: Causes intense and rapid lowering of the blood pressure. This may lead to severe headaches, and even shock-like reactions. Patients should be sitting when inhaling the vapors.
Administration: Inhalation.
Preparations: Dispensed in glass pearls or ampules covered with silk. These are crushed and the vapors inhaled at once.
Dose: 0.3 cc.

AMYLSINE®, see Naepaine

AMYTAL®, see Amobarbital

ANALEPTICS
Amphetamine, Caffeine, Camphor, Ephedrine, Methamphetamine, Nikethamide, Pentylenetetrazole, Picrotoxin, Strychnine.

ANALGESICS
Addictive drugs under federal regulations: Alphaprodine, Codeine, Dihydrocodeine, Dihydrocodeinone, Dihydromorphinone, Ethylmorphine, Meperidine, Methadone, Methorphinan, Metopon, Morphine, Opium, Pantopon®.

Nonaddictive drugs: Acetanilid, Acetophenetidin, Acetyl-para-aminophenol, Acetylsalicylic acid, Aminopyrine, Antipyrine, Carbethyl salicylate, Cinchophen, Dextro propoxyphene, Dipyrone, Methyl salicylate, Neocinchophen, Phenetsal, Phenylbutazone, Salicylamide.

ANAROXYL®, see Carbazochrome Salicylate

ANAYODIN®, see Chiniofon

ANDIRA®, see Pectin

ANDROGENIC HORMONES
Fluoxymestrone, Methyltestosterone, Testosterone.

ANDROLIN®, see Testosterone

ANDRONAQ®, see Testosterone

ANDRONATE®, see Testosterone

ANDRUSOL®, see Testosterone

ANECTINE®, see Succinylcholine

ANESTHESIN®, see Ethyl Aminobenzoate

ANESTHETICS
General: Barbiturates, Chloroform, Cyclopropane, Ether, Ethylene, Ethyl chloride, Hydroxydione, Methurital, Thiopental, Tribromoethanol, Trichloroethylene, Vinyl ether.
Local: Benoxinate, Butethamine, Chloroprocaine, Cocaine, Dibucaine, Dyclonine, Dimethisoquin, Hexylcaine, Lidocaine, Naepaine, Piperocaine, Procaine, Tetracaine.
Surface: Amalone, Butyl aminobenzoate, Chlorobutanol, Clove oil, Cocaine, Cyclomethycaine, Dibucaine, Diperodon, Ethyl aminobenzoate, Menthol, Phenacaine, Piperocaine, Pramoxine, Procaine isobutyrate, Tetracaine.

ANGICAP®, see Pentaerythritol Tetranitrate

ANHYDROHYDROXYPROGESTERONE, see Ethisterone

ANISE OIL
Carminative and flavor. Colorless or pale

ANSADOL

12

yellow oil, with taste and odor of anise.
Soluble in alcohol.
Actions and Uses: Used as a carminative
and for its flavor.
Preparations: Oil, Anise spirit ,10% anise
oil in alcohol. Anise water, saturated solution of the oil in water.

ANSADOL®, see Salicylanilide

ANSOLYSEN®, see Pentolinium

ANTABUSE®, see Disulfiram

ANTACIDS
Aluminum carbonate, Aluminum hydroxide, Aluminum phosphate, Aminoacetic
acid, Bismuth subcarbonate, Calcium
carbonate, Calcium hydroxide, Calcium
oxide, Dihydroxyaluminum aminoacetate,
Magnesia magma, Magnesium carbonate,
Magnesium hydroxide, Magnesium oxide,
Polyamine-methylene resin, Sodium , bicarbonate.

ANTAZOLINE—Antistine®
One of the large group of antihistamine
drugs, which see.

ANTEPAR®, see Piperazine

ANTHALAZINE®, see Piperazine

ANTHRALIN—Cignolin®,
Dithranol®
Dermatologic. Crystalline yellowish
brown powder. Insoluble in water, but
soluble in chloroform and acetone.
Actions and Uses: Stimulates cellular
regeneration and is used in treatment
of psoriasis, and other dermatoses. Not
used internally.
Warnings: May discolor the skin, produce dermatitis or conjunctivitis.
Administration: Topical.
Preparations: Cream or ointment, containing 0.25–0.1% of anthralin in petroleum or aerosol base.
Dose: 0.1–0.25%.

ANTIBIOTICS
General Warning: These are all potent
antibacterial materials and may, especially if used indiscriminately, or for long
periods of time, suppress bacterial
activity which is essential to health; they

may also pave the way for antibiotic-re-
sistant infections, called superinfections.
In addition, pathogenic bacteria may become highly resistant to them. It is essential, therefore, that they be used with
discrimination.
Bacitracin, Carbomycin, Chloramphenicol,
Chlortetracycline, Cycloserine, Dihydrostreptomycin, Erythromycin, Fumagillin,
Gramacidin, Neomycin, Novobiocin, Nystatin, Oleandomycin, Oxytetracycline,
Penicillin, Polymyxin B, Streptomycin,
Tetracycline, Viomycin.

ANTICHOLINERGICS
Atropine, Adiphenine, Aminopentamide,
Amprotropine, Belladonna, Caramiphen,
Cyclopentolate, Cycrimine, Dicyclomine,
Diphemanil, Ethyl-Piperidyl-Benzilate,
Eucatropine, Hexocyclium, Homatropine,
Hyoscine, Hyoscyamine, Methantheline,
Methyl-Piperidyl-Diphenylglycolate, Me-
thscopolamine, Oxyphenonium, Penthien-
ate, Pipenzolate, Piperidolate, Procycli-
dine, Propantheline, Scopolamine, Tri-
cyclamol, Tridihexide, Trihexyphenidyl.

ANTICOAGULANTS
Acenocoumarin, Bishydroxycoumarin,
Cyclocumarol, Diphenadione, Ethyl Biscoumacetate, Heparin, Phenindione, Warfarin.

ANTICONVULSANTS
Barbiturate: Mephobarbital, Metharbital,
Phenobarbital.
Reduced Barbiturate: Mysoline.
Hydantoinate: Diphenylhydantoin, Etho-
toin, Methylphenylethylhydantoin.
Oxazolidine: Paramethadione, Trimetha-
dione.
Curariform: Chondodendron Tomentosum
Extract, Dimethyl-tubocurarine, Galla-
mine, Succinylcholine, Tubocurarine.
Phenacetylurea: Phenaceamide.
Miscellaneous: Methylphenylsuccinimide.

ANTIHISTAMINICS
Used to relieve or prevent allergic symptoms. They provide only symptomatic
relief and their action never extends beyond the few hours of the duration of
their effects. They are not curative.

There is the danger of toxic action, especially drowsiness after many of them, and the patient should be warned. Often one of these drugs may be found which is both effective and nontoxic for the patient; often one member is far more effective or less toxic for the patient than any of the others. There is no way of predicting, for a particular patient, which member of the group will prove to be the most desirable. More recently certain of the antihistaminic drugs have been found useful for the relief of nausea and vomiting and motion sickness. Many of these drugs exert fairly potent sedative actions and, because it is legal to sell antihistaminics without prescription, one of these, methapyrilene, is being sold under a variety of names, such as Dormin®, for sedative purposes.

Antazoline, Bromodiphenlhydramine, Buclizine, Chlorcyclizine, Chlorothen, Chlorpromazine, Chlorprophenpyridamine, Cyclizine, Dimenhydrinate, Diphenhydramine, Diphenylpyraline, Doxylamine, Meclizine, Methapheniline, Methapyrilene, Paracarbinoxamine, Phenyltoloxamine, Promethazine, Prophenpyridamine, Pyrilamine, Pyrithiazine, Pyrrobutamine, Thonzylamine, Tripelennamine.

ANTI-INFLAMMATORY DRUGS
Antipyrine derivatives, Anti-inflammatory hormones, Cinchophen, Chymotrypsin, Colchicine, Neo-cinchophen, Phenylbutazone, Salicylates, Trypsin.

ANTI-INFLAMMATORY HORMONES
Corticotropin, Cortisone, Hydrocortamate, Fludrocortisone, Methylprednisolone, Prednisolone, Prednisone.

ANTILUETICS
It should be noted that, as matters stand, penicillin is, far and away, the drug of choice and heavy metals, arsenic and bismuth are now largely of historic interest and useful occasionally in very unusual situations.

ANTIMONY
Most of the antimony compounds used in medicine are chemotherapeutic agents against tropical disease, especially of protozoan origin. Tartar emetic, not only has this use, but is sometimes used as a nauseant expectorant and an emetic. Many preparations are given by the parenteral route only. All antimony compounds are potentially toxic and cumulative and should be used with caution. The antidote for antimony is not well established, but it may be well to try dimercaprol.

Antimony potassium tartrate, Antimony sodium thioglycollate, Ethylstibamine, Stibamine glucoside, Stibophen.

ANTIMONY POTASSIUM TARTRATE—Tartar Emetic
Expectorant, antiprotozoal and emetic. Colorless, transparent crystals or white powder. Soluble in water.

Absorption: Slowly absorbed from G. I. tract. Eliminated by kidneys in about 3 days.

Actions and Uses: Orally in small doses, it may be used as an expectorant. Much more frequently used, by intravenous injection, in the management of granuloma inguinale and schistosomiasis. There is a question whether it may be of value in the treatment of trichinosis.

Warnings: Extravasation during intravenous injection may cause painful reaction due to irritant nature of drug. Drug may cause nausea, vomiting, stiffness, epigastric pain, constrictive sensation in chest, slow cardiac rate, dizziness, collapse. Should not be used in the presence of severe heart, liver or kidney disease. Should not be used together with other heavy metals.

Administration: Oral, intravenous.

Preparations: Expectorant. Ampule, solution for injection, 1.0%.

Dose: Expectorant, 3 mg. Parenteral, 30 mg.

Antidote: Not established but it is well to try dimercaprol.

ANTIMONY SODIUM THIOGLYCOLLATE
Chemotherapeutic. White or pink powder, usually odorless, discolored by exposure to light. Soluble in water.

Actions and Uses: Less toxic and irritant than antimony potassium tartrate, and proposed as a substitute for it in the treatment of tropical diseases. Not given orally. Eliminated by the kidneys.
Warnings: Same as for antimony potassium tartrate.
Administration: Intramuscular.
Preparations: Powder. Ampule, 0.5% solution in 10 and 20 cc. sized ampules.
Dose: 50 mg.
Antidote: Not established but it is well to try dimercaprol.

ANTIPRURITICS
Anesthetics (surface), Camphor, Clove oil, Crotamiton, Menthol, Phenol, Sodium bicarbonate, Starch.

ANTIPYRETICS
Acetanilid, Acetylsalicylic acid, Acetophenetidin, Aminopyrine, Antipyrine, Cinchophen, Methyl salicylate, Neo-cinchophen, Quinine, Sodium salicylate.

ANTIPYRINE—Phenazone
Analgesic and antipyretic. Colorless crystals or white powder. Soluble in water.
Actions and Uses: Chemically and pharmacologically much the same as aminopyrine. Rarely used.
Warnings: Same as aminopyrine.
Administration: Oral.
Preparations: Tablet.
Dose: 0.3 Gm.

ANTISEPTICS
Intestinal: Antibiotics, Sulfonamides.
Local: Aminitrozole, Antibiotics, Alcohol (ethyl and iso-propyl), Acetomeroctol, Ammoniated mercury, Bacitracin, Benzalkonium, Benzethonium, Bismuth tribromophenate, Carbamide Peroxide, Carbolfuchsin, Cetyl pyridinium, Chloroazodin, Coal tar, Cresol, Furazolidone, Halazone, Hexetidine, Hydrogen peroxide, Ichthammol, Iodine, Merbromin, Mercury bichloride, Methylbenzethonium, Methylrosaniline, Neomycin, Nitromersol, Nitrofurazone, Phenol, Pine tar, Polymyxin B, Providone-Iodine, Potassium permanganate, Pyrethrum, Resorcinol, Salicylic acid, Silver chloride, Silver iodide, Silver picrate, Silver protein, Sodium perborate, Sulfur, Thimerosal, Thymol, Turpentine oil, Tyrothricin, Zinc peroxide.
Urinary: Acriflavine, Ammonium mandelate, Antibiotics, Methenamine, Methylene blue, Nitrofurantoin, Phenylazodiamino-pyridine, Silver nitrate, Silver protein, Sulfonamides.

ANTISEPTIC SOLUTION—Liquor Antisepticus
Antiseptic. A solution containing boric acid (2.5%), aromatic oils, alcohol (25%) and water. Characteristic aromatic odor. Becomes cloudy on extreme cold, but is clear and colorless at normal room temperatures.
Actions and Uses: A pleasant mouth wash when diluted with 3-5 parts of water. Not used internally. Has little antiseptic value.
Warnings: Must be diluted before using.
Administration: Topical, gargle with diluted solution and expectorate.

ANTISPASMODICS
Intestinal: Anticholinergic drugs.
Respiratory: Adrenergic drugs, Aminophylline, Potassium iodide, Stramonium.
Skeletal: See muscle relaxants.

ANTISTINE®, see Antazoline

ANTRENYL®, see Oxyphenonium

APAMIDE®, see Acetyl-para-aminophenol

APOMORPHINE
Emetic. White or grayish powder or crystals, usually the hydrochloride. Soluble in water. Solutions change color, from gray to green to black on standing.
Actions and Uses: Produces vomiting by an action on the brain. Used when effective vomiting is quickly needed, as in poisoning. Effects produced within 5 minutes after injection and may be long lasting.
Warnings: Excessive vomiting. Solutions which are green must not be used. Considered a narcotic and under control of federal law.
Administration: Subcutaneous.

15 ASPIDIUM OLEORESIN

Preparations: Hypo tablet, 5 mg. Solution. Solutions deteriorate on standing. Keep in dark.
Dose: Usually about 5 mg. for an adult, subcutaneously. If the first does not produce an effect, subsequent doses may cause central depression without producing vomiting.

APRESOLINE®, see Hydralazine

APRICOT KERNEL OIL, see Persic Oil

APROBARBITAL—Alurate®
One of the intermediate acting barbiturates, which see.

AQUA FORTIS, see Nitric Acid, Fuming

ARACHIS OIL, see Peanut oil

ARALEN®, see Chloroquine

ARAMINE®, see Metaraminol

ARANTHOLE®, see Methylamino-hydroxy-methylheptane

ARGYROL®, see Silver Protein

ARISTOCORT®, see Triamcinolone

ARISTOL®, see Thymol Iodide

ARLIDIN®, see Nylidrin

ARMAZIDE®, see Isoniazid

AROMATIC SPIRIT OF AMMONIA, see Ammonia

ARSENIC
Arsenic compounds are widely used in medicine. They have been particularly useful in diseases caused by protozoa, although they have been used in noninfectious disease as well, especially skin and blood dyscrasias. All have serious toxic potentialities and those receiving arsenicals must be carefully watched. BAL (dimercaprol) should be used as the antidote for all forms of arsenic poisoning. In syphilis it has been virtually entirely displaced by penicillin.
Acetarsone, Arsenic Trioxide, Arsphenamine, Arsthinol, Bismuth Arsphenamine, Glycobiarsol, Carbarsone, Dichlorophenarsine, Oxophenarsine, Phenarsone, Potassium Arsenite, Sodium Cacodylate, Tryparsamide.

ARSENIC TRIOXIDE
Hematinic. White powder, slightly soluble in water.
Actions and Uses: Occasionally used in the treatment of leukemia to depress white cell formation. Used in some skin diseases.
Warnings: An extremely toxic material; may cause serious kidney damage.
Administration: Oral, topical.
Preparations: Solution, 1% in about 5% hydrochloric acid. Tablet, 2 mg.
Dose: 2 mg. for the adult.
Antidote for all arsenicals: Dimercaprol.

ARSPHENAMINE—Salvarsan®, 606
Antiluetic. The original antisyphilitic arsenical; now completely replaced by such modern arsenicals as oxophenarsine and penicillin. See Arsenic.

ARSTHINOL—Balarsen®
An organic arsenical for oral use in intestinal amebiasis and yaws. See arsenic.
Antidote: Dimercaprol.

ARTANE®, see Trihexyphenidyl

ARTERENOL, see Levarterenol

ASCORBIC ACID—Cevitamic Acid, Cebione®, Cevex®, Vitamin C.
Cevitamic Acid, Cebione®, Cevex®, Vitamin C.
Vitamin. White or yellowish powder, soluble in water. Solution deteriorates rapidly. Sodium salt available.
Actions and Uses: Essential element of diet. Not stored in body to any extent and is needed regularly in the diet. Lack of this vitamin for a period of time may produce scurvy or less severe evidences of vitamin C deficiency, such as prolonged healing of wounds.
Warnings: Large doses may lead to G. I. upsets.
Administration: Oral, intramuscular, intravenous.
Preparations: Tablet, 25, 50, 100 mg. Ampule; sodium ascorbate solution usually used for parenteral administration.
Dose: Depends on needs of the patient.

ASPIDIUM OLEORESIN—Male Fern Oleoresin

Vermifuge. The oleoresin, a dark green thick liquid, insoluble in water.
Actions and Uses: Toxic to the tapeworm and used in treatment of tapeworm infestations. Also toxic to host in large doses.
Warnings: If absorbed, may cause violent symptoms: vomiting, purging, weakness, spasm of extremities, convulsions, stupor, coma, collapse, permanent blindness, jaundice and kidney damage. Should not be used in debilitated patients, those with cardiac, liver, or kidney disease, ulcerative lesions of G. I. tract. A second course should not be given within a week of the first.
Administration: Oral. A fat-free diet should be given for 48 hours before the drug, and a liquid diet 24 hours before. Two hours after the drug, a saline purgative is given, and 2 hours later, a soap solution enema. 15-30 Gm. sodium sulfate given night before the drug. Castor oil and mineral oil are contraindicated.
Preparations: Capsule, Emulsion.
Dose: Two doses of 2.5 Gm. of the oleoresin given 1 hour apart in the morning, followed as above with purgative and enema.

ASPIRIN, see Acetylsalicylic Acid

ASPOGEN®, see Dihydroxyaluminum Aminoacetate

ASTEROL®, see Diamthazole

ASTRINGENTS
Alcohol, Aluminum salts, Ammonia, Cupric sulfate, Iodine, Mercuric chloride, Mustard, Nitric acid, Phenol, Salicylic acid, Silver nitrate, Tannic acid, Zinc salts.

ATABRINE®, see Quinacrine

ATARACTICS, see Tranquilizers

ATARAX®, see Hydroxyzine

ATOPHAN®, see Cinchophen

ATROPINE
Anticholinergic and mydriatic. A white crystalline material obtained from belladonna; the active principle of belladonna.

Extremely bitter. Alkaloid is insoluble; the sulfate is quite soluble in water.
Absorption: Well absorbed from G. I. tract, the surface of the eye, or after injection.
Actions and Uses: Atropine is prototype of vagal antagonists. It paralyses or depresses the vagus and the other nerves of the parasympathetic nervous system. By this action, it depresses salivation, the secretion of gastric juices and acid, and pancreatic juices. It suppresses the secretion of bronchial mucous membranes. It relaxes muscles which contract under vagal tone, thus it relaxes bronchial musculature, the smooth muscle of the intestine, and dilates the pupils. It suppresses perspiration and accelerates the heart. It is used in the treatment of spasm of the G. I. tract, bronchial spasm, in peptic ulcer to suppress gastric secretion and activity, before anesthesia to keep the bronchial secretions at a minimum. The rate of elimination varies with different organs.
Warnings: Overdosage may lead to elevated temperature and delirium. The prolonged effect on the pupil may be overcome with physostigmine. Mouth may become uncomfortably dry. In patients with glaucoma or a tendency to it, it may cause extremely painful acute glaucoma with loss of sight. For this reason atropine is rarely applied to the eyes of patients over 45, and used with special caution by mouth. This warning applies to all atropine-like drugs.
Administration: Oral, parenteral, topical (in eye).
Preparations: Tincture of belladonna. Tablet, triturate. Solution, for injection. Discs, to be placed directly on the conjunctiva.
Dose: Average adult dose, 0.5 mg.

AU^{198}, see Radio-Gold Colloid

AUREOMYCIN®, see Chlortetracycline

AUROTHIOGLUCOSE—Solganal®
A gold salt used in the treatment of rheumatoid arthritis. See Gold.

AUROTHIOGLYCANIDE—
Lauron®
A gold salt used in the treatment of rheumatoid arthritis. See Gold.

AUTONOMIC DRUGS
Adrenergic, sympathomimetic.
Adrenolytic, sympatholytic.
Anticholinergic, parasympatholytic, vagolytic.
Cholinergic, parasympathomimetic, vagomimetic.

AVERTIN®, see Tribromoethanol

AVLOSULFON®, see Diaminodiphenylsulfone

AZACYCLONAL—Frenquel®
Tranquilizer.
Actions and Uses: New agent used to prevent schizophrenic hallucinations and, in many ways, to induce quiescence in hyperactive states although stated not to be a sedative.
Warnings: New drug not yet clearly evaluated; addiction potention not established.
Administration: Oral.
Preparations: 20 mg. tablets (blue).
Dose: 20 mg. three times a day.

AZAPETINE—Ilidar®
Adrenolytic, vasodilator.
Actions and Uses: Antagonizes sympathetic constriction of blood vessels and vasoconstrictor action of epinephrine, and, in addition, claimed to relax blood vessels by direct action. Used in vascular disease with vasospasm, Raynaud's Syndrome, phlebitis, etc. As with other drugs in the group, of limited utility.
Warnings: May cause intense fall in blood pressure. Do not use in anginal syndrome or other form of coronary disease, asthma, or peptic ulcer.
Administration: Oral.
Preparations: Tablets, 25 mg.
Dose: 25 mg. three times daily.

AZOCHLORAMID®, see Chloroazodin

AZULFIDINE®, see Salicylazosulfapyridine

B

BACITRACIN—Ginebatin®, Parentracin®, Topitracin®
Antibiotic. Obtained from *Bacillus subtilis.*
Actions and Uses: Effective against many common pus-forming bacteria. Used only topically.
Warnings: Very toxic systemically; use only topically.
Administration: Topical.
Preparations: Powder, ointment, suppository.
Dose: Units; concentration depends on site of administration, usually about 500 Units per Gm.

BAKING SODA, see Sodium Bicarbonate

BAL, see Dimercaprol

BALARSEN®, see Arsthinol

BALSAM OF PERU
Antiseptic, epithelial stimulant.
Actions and Uses: An ointment used in treatment of indolent ulcers, mildly stimulating cell proliferation. Also used in treatment of fungus infections of skin and skin infections of other types.
Warnings: Stains from these ointments are exceedingly difficult to remove from linen. Store ointment in a cool place.
Administration: Topical.
Preparations: Ointment.
Dose: Concentration, 10% with a bland base.

BANTHINE®, see Methantheline

BANTRON®, see Lobeline

BARBITAL—Medinal®, Veronal®
Hypnotic. White crystals.
Actions and Uses: Barbital is the most slowly acting of all the members of this group, and in many cases may lead to a "hang-over" in the morning following a dose.
Warnings: As for other barbiturates.
Administration: Oral.
Preparations: Tablet and capsule.
Dose: 0.15-0.5 Gm.
Antidote: Picrotoxin.

BARBITONE®, see Barbital

BARBITURATES

There is a long list of compounds which are derived from the original drug, barbital, and in general, share its properties and dangers. In general, the barbiturates are very insoluble in the acid form and very soluble as the sodium salt.

These are all synthetic compounds, the acid form is insoluble in water, the sodium salts are very soluble. They are bitter and relatively well absorbed from G. I. tract but vary considerably in the rate of absorption and the speed of development of effects. Similarly, they vary in rate of elimination. In general, those with rapid onset of action are also relatively rapidly eliminated; those slow to produce effects produce the more longlasting effects. In general, too, the rapidly eliminated drugs are destroyed in part or all in the liver, those with longlasting effects are eliminated by the kidneys in the urine.

Each of the barbiturates may produce sedation, hypnosis, somnolence and surgical anesthesia depending on the dose given.

The drugs are commonly used as sedatives and for the relief of insomnia. The more rapidly acting ones like thiopental, may be used for surgical anesthesia. Phenobarbital seems to have special effects against the convulsions of epilepsy not possessed by the other members of the group.

Continued use may lead to resistance and dependence. Withdrawal symptoms, such as convulsions and anxiety, may develop if drugs are suddenly stopped after long continued use. Alcoholics may substitute barbiturates for alcohol, and become just as devoted to it. The effects are similar. Overdosage may lead to profound narcosis, respiratory depression and death. Barbiturates are presently the favorite drug for suicide. Poisoning is usually effectively treated with supportive therapy alone. Penicillin should be used to prevent pneumonia. Shock may develop and require the standard treatment. In rare cases which do not respond to these measures, analeptics such as picrotoxin, in the hands of the expert only, may sometimes be an effective measure.

Available in tablets, capsules, suppositories and solution for parenteral administration.

Dosage varies somewhat with each drug. It is to be noted, however, that the therapeutic index for all is about the same: drugs which require the smallest dose to produce therapeutic effects, also are the most toxic; those which have larger therapeutic doses are also less toxic.

Very rapid acting: Hexobarbital, Thiamylal, Thiopental.

Rapid acting: Allylbarbital, Butallylonal, Cyclobarbital, Heptabarbital, Hexethal, Pentobarbital, Secobarbital, Talbutal.

Intermediate acting: Amobarbital, Aprobarbital, Butabarbital, Butethal, Diallylbarbital, Probarbital, Vinbarbital.

Long acting: Barbital, Mephobarbital, Phenobarbital.

BARIUM CHLORIDE

Actions and Uses: Rarely used today. Formerly used in treatment of heart block.

Warnings: An extremely dangerous drug.

BARIUM SULFATE

Diagnostic. A fine white powder, insoluble in water. Has chalky taste. Mixed with water, it makes a paste.

Absorption: Not absorbed from G. I. tract and passes unchanged through it.

Actions and Uses: Barium sulfate is opaque to x-rays. Drug is taken by mouth for x-rays of upper part of G.I. tract, and given as a "barium enema" to outline the rectum and colon.

Warnings: When taken by mouth in large amounts, unless the bowels move and evacuate actively, impaction may form. There is the danger of confusion of barium sulfate with other barium salts which are extremely toxic.

Administration: Oral, rectal.

Preparations: The thickness of the paste required depends on the kind of roentgenology. A very thin mixture is gen-

19

erally used, but in instances in which the esophagus is to be outlined, a thick paste may be desirable.
Dose: As indicated by needs.

BASALJEL®, see Aluminum Carbonate

BASEX®, see Polyamine-methylene Resins

BAY OIL, see Myrcia Oil

BELLADONNA
Anticholinergic. Powdered leaf of the plant, *Atropa belladonna.* Has bitter taste.
Actions and Uses: Its actions and uses depend on the fact that it contains atropine and a related alkaloid, with similar actions, hyoscyamine. Used mainly in the relief of spasm of the intestinal musculature and in peptic ulcer.
Warnings: Overdosage may lead to mydriasis, dryness of mouth, elevated temperature and delirium. Rarely fatal. May cause glaucoma.
Administration: Oral.
Preparations: Extract, fluidextract and tincture. Alkaloidal mixture (Rabellon®).
Dose: The equivalent of 0.06 Gm. of the leaf, i.e., 0.6 cc. of the tincture.
Antidote: Physostigmine.

BENACTYZINE—Suavitil®
Tranquilizer. New drug, and like all new tranquilizers it will take a long time before its usefulness in the treatment of simple anxiety symptoms will be established. Available in 1 mg. tablets.

BENADRYL®, see Diphenhydramine

BENEMID®, see Probenecid

BENODAINE®, see Piperoxan

BENOQUIN®, see Monobenzone

BENOXINATE—Dorsacaine®
Local anesthetic. Used largely in opthalmology. A few drops of an 0.4% solution applied to the eye will usually provide adequate surface anesthesia very promptly. Use cautiously in patients with a history of allergic reactions, with open lesions, or heart disease.

BENTONITE
Emulsifying agent. A fine buff or cream-colored powder, insoluble in water, but swelling considerably when added to it.
Actions and Uses: An adsorbent, emulsifying, gel-forming material used in the preparation of pharmaceuticals and cosmetics. Also a detergent but rarely used as such.

BENTYL®, see Dicyclomine

BENYLATE®, see Benzyl benzoate

BENZALKONIUM—Zephiran®
Antiseptic. A soluble powder with an aromatic odor and a bitter taste.
Actions and Uses: Cationic detergent and surface active material with disinfectant properties in high dilution, with little irritant properties for man. Its antibacterial action is exerted relatively rapidly, within about 5 minutes.
Warnings: Effectiveness is antagonized by soaps. In high concentration irritant to skin and mucous membranes.
Administration: Topical.
Preparations: Solution, from 1:1000 to 1:20,000.
Dose: Concentration depends on surface to be treated.

BENZATHINE PENICILLIN G—
Bicillin®, Neolin®, Permapen®
Antibiotic. Relatively stable at room temperature.
Actions and Uses: Same uses as procaine penicillin but with considerably longer action. See Penicillin.
Warnings: Same as for penicillin, which see.
Administration: Intramuscular, oral.
Preparations: Oral suspension, tablet and suspension for injection.
Dose: 300,000–600,000 Units.

BENZEDREX®, see Propylhexedrine

BENZEDRINE®, see Amphetamine

BENZENE—Benzol
Solvent. Never used in medicinal preparations.
Warnings: Inflammable. Extremely toxic;

may lead to serious depression of bone marrow.

BENZENE HEXACHLORIDE, GAMMA—Gexane®, Kwell®

Parasiticide. White crystals, insoluble in water.
Actions and Uses: In treatment of scabies and pediculosis.
Warnings: Excessive amounts applied to the skin may be absorbed and produce toxic effects.
Administration: Topical.
Preparations: Solution, 1%. Ointment, 1%.
Dose: Up to 1% concentration.

BENZESTROL

Synthetic estrogen. Not a stilbestrol derivative. Available in liquid preparations and 0.5-5 mg. tablets. Dosage of the order of 2-3 mg. daily orally for menopausal symptoms. See Estrogens.

BENZETHONIUM—Phemerol®

Antiseptic. The chloride. A general antiseptic used for preoperative preparations as well as for general purposes. Available in 3% and 0.1% solution, and 0.2% tincture; the latter two concentrations are recommended for general antiseptic purposes.

BENZOCAINE®, see Ethyl Aminobenzoate

BENZOIC ACID

Antiseptic. White crystals.
Absorption: Well absorbed from G. I. tract.
Actions and Uses: Little effect if taken in small dosage by mouth. Has only mild antiseptic action. Commonly used together with salicylic acid in an ointment called Whitfield's ointment, for the treatment of fungus infections of the skin.
Administration: Topical.
Preparations: Ointment, commonly combined in 12% strength with salicylic acid 6% to form Whitfield's ointment.

BENZOIN

Antiseptic. Aromatic resin with acrid taste.
Actions and Uses: Used as local anti-

septic and stimulant to promote healing. Used in inhalations as an expectorant.
Warnings: Some feel that benzoin, which is most frequently used in steam inhalations for irritations and inflammation in the tracheo-bronchial tree, may cause more irritation than good. When used for this purpose, the vapors should smell only slightly of the benzoin.
Administration: Topical, steam inhalation.
Preparations: Compound tincture of benzoin, contains about 10% of the resin.
Dose: As indicated.

BENZOL, see Benzene

BENZTROPINE—Cogentin®

Skeletal muscle relaxant. Combines atropine-like action with antihistaminic and local anesthetic properties. Usefulness of this diffuse action not established. May have sedative action, as well. Suggested for paralysis agitans. Dosage of the order of 1 or 2 mg. daily.

BENZPYRINIUM—Stigmonene®

Cholinergic. White or yellowish powder, the bromide, soluble in water.
Actions and Uses: A cholinergic drug with much the same actions, effects and uses as physostigmine and neostigmine.
Warnings: May cause nausea or vomiting, slow heart rate, hypotension, or induce asthmatic reaction. Do not use in mechanical intestinal obstruction.
Administration: Parenteral.
Preparations: Ampule.
Dose: 0.5 mg.
Antidote: Atropine.

BENZYL ALCOHOL—Phenylcarbinol

Surface anesthetic. Clear fluid miscible with water.
Actions and Uses: Used for its local anesthetic actions in the control of pruritis.
Warnings: Toxic by mouth.
Administration: Topical.
Preparations: Usually with other drugs.
Dose: Concentration 1-4%.

BENZYL BENZOATE—Benylate®, Vanzoate®

Scabicide. A clear colorless, oily liquid

with aromatic odor and sharp burning taste. Insoluble in water.
Actions and Uses: Originally used as an antispasmodic, an action which cannot be depended upon. Has recently been shown effective in treatment of scabies and pediculosis.
Warnings: Do not apply to face or near eyes.
Administration: Topical.
Preparations: Lotion and lotion with chlorophenothane (DDT).
Dose: Concentration, about 10% benzyl benzoate.

BETADINE®, see Povidone-Iodine

BETA-PYRIDYL CARBINOL—Roniacol®
Vasodilator. The tartrate. Recommended for vasospastic conditions and other conditions with deficient peripheral blood supply.
Preparations: Tablet, 50 mg. Solution, 50 mg. per teaspoonful.
Dose: Ranges from 50-200 mg., 1-4 times daily.

BETAZOLE—Histalog®
Analogue of histamine; said to stimulate the secretion of hydrochloric acid without fall in blood pressure which may follow histamine. Substitute for histamine in gastric analysis. Dose is usually of the order of 50 mg.

BETHANECHOL—Urecholine®
Cholinergic. White powder, the chloride, soluble in water.
Actions and Uses: Much the same as methacholine but with somewhat more persistent actions. Used mainly in intestinal stasis, abdominal distention and urinary retention.
Warnings: Hypotension and substernal distress may sometimes follow injection. Keep atropine at hand when using drug.
Administration: Subcutaneous, oral.
Preparations: Tablet, 5 mg. Ampule, 5 mg. in 1 cc.
Dose: 2.5-10 mg.
Antidote: Atropine.

BEVIDOX®, see Vitamin B_{12}

BIALLYLAMICOL—Camoform®
Amebicide. Recently introduced. Dosage of the order of 500 mg. three times a day. About 10 percent of patients report some kind of side effect.

BICILLIN®, see Benzathine Penicillin G

BIEBRICH SCARLET RED, see Scarlet Red

BILE SALTS, see Ox Bile Extract

BILRON®, see Iron Bile Salts

BIOLOGICALS
Biologicals are materials elaborated by living organisms, usually bacteria or animals. Biologicals should be carefully examined for description of their use, instruction on storage, expiration date, and allergies (especially in the case of egg-medium viruses, etc.). These include Antitoxins, Serums, Toxins, Toxoids, Vaccines. Very few of these preparations are described here.

BIO-SORB®, see Starch-derivative Dusting Powder

BISHYDROXYCOUMARIN —Dicumarol®
Anticoagulant. White crystalline powder with slightly bitter taste. Insoluble in water.
Absorption: Well absorbed from G. I. tract, producing full effects within 12-24 hours after oral administration and persisting for about 72 hours.
Actions and Uses: Lengthens prothrombin time by decreasing prothrombin content of blood, preventing intravascular clotting and propagation of emboli and thrombi. Used mainly in patients with coronary thrombosis to prevent intramural thrombi, in patients with thrombophlebitis and in prevention of emboli.
Warnings: Overdosage may lead to internal hemorrhage. Drug must be used in conjunction with daily prothrombin tests which determine the dose for the day. In overdosage, intravenous injection of vitamin K or menadione and transfusions of fresh whole blood may restore normal prothrombin content of the blood.

Administration: Oral.
Preparations: Tablet and capsule, 25, 50, 100 mg.
Dose: Depends on results of daily prothrombin test and intensity of effects desired. Dosage varies greatly from patient to patient.
Antidote: Vitamin K, fresh whole blood transfusion.

BISMARSEN®, see Bismuth Arsphenamine

BISMUTH
Two groups of bismuth compounds: (1) Insoluble compounds, usually the basic "sub" salts of bismuth which are used for mechanical protection of irritated or inflamed surfaces, the skin and mucous membranes. Absorption from G. I. tract usually negligible. Often used in treatment of diarrhea and also, because of buffering action, as antacids. (2) Other bismuth salts which are fairly potent against the spirochete and were alternated with the arsenical drugs when the arsenicals were used in syphilis. Bismuth may cause toxic effects: skin eruptions, stomatitis and renal irritation.
Bismuth Arsphenamine, Bismuth Ethylcamphorate, Bismuth Potassium Tartrate, Bismuth Sodium Tartrate, Bismuth Sodium Triglycollamate, Bismuth Subcarbonate, Bismuth Subgallate, Bismuth Subnitrate, Bismuth Subsalicylate, Bismuth Thioglycollate, Bismuth Tribromophenate, Glycobiarsol, Sodium Iodobismuthite.

BISMUTH ARSPHENAMINE
—Bismarsen®
Antiluetic. Largely replaced in treatment of syphilis by penicillin and little used at present.

BISMUTH ETHYLCAMPHORATE
Antiluetic. Rarely used mainly because replaced by penicillin.

BISMUTH POTASSIUM TARTRATE
Antiluetic. White powder with sweetish taste. Soluble in water.
Absorption: Rapidly absorbed from intramuscular injection.
Actions and Uses: May be given in con-

junction with arsenicals for treatment of syphilis, but largely replaced by penicillin. A mild diuretic. See bismuth.

BISMUTH SODIUM TARTRATE
Antiluetic. Largely replaced by penicillin in treatment of syphilis.

BISMUTH SODIUM THIOGLYCOLLATE—Thio-Bismol®
Antiluetic. Largely replaced by penicillin in treatment of syphilis.

BISMUTH SODIUM TRIGLYCOLLAMATE—Bistrimate®
Antileutic. Largely replaced by penicillin in treatment of syphilis.

BISMUTH SUBCARBONATE
Protective and antacid. White or yellowish-white powder, insoluble in water.
Absorption: Not appreciably absorbed from G. I. tract.
Actions and Uses: Used internally and externally as protectant in wounds and ulcers, and to neutralize gastric acidity. An emollient in gastritis, enteritis, etc.
Warnings: May lead to constipation. Absorption may occur with toxic effects. See Bismuth.
Administration: Oral, topical.
Preparations: Tablet and powder.
Dose: 1–5 Gm.

BISMUTH SUBGALLATE
Absorbent and protective. Bright yellow powder, insoluble in water.
Absorption: Not appreciably absorbed from G. I. tract.
Actions and Uses: Same as bismuth subcarbonate, but has no antacid action.
Warnings: Same as the subcarbonate.
Administration: Oral.
Preparations: Tablet and powder.
Dose: 0.5–2.0 Gm.

BISMUTH SUBNITRATE
Protective. White powder, insoluble in water.
Absorption: Significant amounts may be absorbed from wounds and G. I. tract.
Actions and Uses: Same as bismuth subcarbonate, but has no antacid actions.
Warnings: May yield nitrite and produce nitrite poisoning. After large doses, it

may be absorbed in sufficient amount to produce bismuth poisoning.

Administration: Topical, oral (seldom).
Preparations: Tablet, powder and ointment.
Dose: 1 Gm.

BISMUTH SUBSALICYLATE
Antiluetic. Largely replaced by penicillin.

BISMUTH TRIBROMOPHENATE —Xeroform®
Antiseptic. White powder.
Actions and Uses: Nonirritating antiseptic used in skin infections and dressing skin wounds.
Warnings: Local reactions in sensitive cases.
Administration: Topical.
Preparations: Ointment, powder and powder filled gauze.
Dose: Concentration, 5%.

BISTRIUM®, see Hexamethonium

BITHIONOL—Lorothidol®
Antiseptic used mainly in soap.

BITTER ALMOND OIL, see Almond Oil, Bitter

BITTER ORANGE OIL
Aromatic flavor.
Actions and Uses: A flavoring agent.

BLAUD'S PILLS, see Ferrous Carbonate

BLUE VITRIOL, see Cupric Sulfate

BLUTENE®, see Tolonium

BONAMINE®, see Meclizine

BORIC ACID
Antiseptic. White or colorless crystals, soluble in water.
Absorption: Well absorbed from G. I. tract.
Actions and Uses: Mild antiseptic in skin and ocular infections.
Warnings: Serious and fatal accidents have occurred from internal use and parenteral administration.
Administration: Topical.
Preparations: Ointment, solution and dusting powder.
Dose: Concentrations, 2–5%.

BORNATE®, see Isobornyl Thiocyanoacetate

BRANDY, see Alcohol

BREWER'S YEAST, see Vitamin B Complex

BRILLIANT GREEN
Antiseptic and epithelial stimulant. A green dye soluble in water.
Actions and Uses: An antiseptic dye. Stimulant to epithelialization.
Warnings: Stains linens.
Administration: Topical.
Preparations: Solution in water.
Dose: Concentration, 0.2%

BRISTAMIN®, see Phenyltoloxamine

BRITISH ANTI-LEWISITE, see Dimercaprol

BROMIDES
The bromides have been long and widely used for sedation and hypnosis. They are slowly eliminated and may cumulate. As a consequence, toxic symptoms tend to develop insidiously in continuous users. Skin eruptions are common. More important, however, is the development of serious psychologic symptoms. Bromides are frequently incorporated into remedies sold over the drug counter without prescription and as a result, poisoning is relatively common. Federal restrictions have reduced the doses of bromides permitted in such remedies.

The value of bromides as sedatives is questionable, and in view of this, use is slowly being eliminated; many hospital formularies have omitted them.

Bromide poisoning is treated by administration of large amounts of sodium chloride. There is no difference in action or potency between the various bromides available.

BROMISOVALUM—Bromural®
Sedative. White tasteless crystals, barely soluble in water.
Actions and Uses: A sedative of moderately long action, not belonging to the barbiturate group. Infrequently used.
Warnings: The same as for all sedatives, dependence may develop.

Administration: Oral.
Preparations: Powder. Tablet, 0.3 Gm.
Dose: 0.3 to 0.6 Gm.

BROMODIPHENHYDRAMINE—
Ambodryl®
An antihistaminic, which see.

BROMSULPHALEIN®, see Sulfo-
bromophthalein

BROMURAL®, see Bromisovalum

BRONKEKPHRINE®, see
Ethylnorepinephrine

BRUCINE
Archaic drug, having properties and dangers similar to those of strychnine.

BUCLIZINE—Vibazine®
Antihistaminic, anti-emetic. Final therapeutic position remains to be established. Available in 50 mg. tablets.

BUROW'S SOLUTION, see Aluminum Acetate

BURSOLINE®, see Diglycocoll Hydroiodide-Iodine

BUSULFAN—Myleran®
Bone-marrow depressant. Tends to act selectively on granulocytes. In large doses, however, thrombocytes, erythocytes and lymphocytes are also depressed. Recommended, therefore, for granulocytic leukemias. Administered orally, in doses ranging from 2 to 6 mg. daily. There is danger from bleeding, agranulocytosis, and generalized bone-marrow depression.

BUTABARBITAL—Butisol®
One of the intermediate acting barbiturates, which see.

BUTACAINE—Butyn®
Surface anesthetic. White crystalline powder, soluble in water.
Actions and Uses: Anesthetic, used for local anesthesia in the eye, nose and throat.
Warnings: Excessive amounts applied topically, especially to broken skin, may be absorbed with toxic effects
Administration: Topical.
Preparations: Solution.
Dose: Concentration, 2%.

BUTALLYLONAL—Pernoston®
One of the rapid acting barbiturates, which see.

BUTAZOLIDIN®, see Phenylbutazone

BUTESIN®, see Butyl Aminobenzoate

BUTETHAL—Neonal®
One of the intermediate acting barbiturates, which see.

BUTETHAMINE—Monocaine®
Local anesthetic. White powder, the formate or hydrochloride, soluble in water.
Actions and Uses: Much the same as procaine but somewhat more potent and toxic.
Warnings: See Procaine.

BUTISOL®, see Butabarbital

BUTYL AMINOBENZOATE—
Butesin®
Surface anesthetic. White powder, almost insoluble in water.
Actions and Uses: Local anesthetic with prolonged effects. Suitable for topical administration.
Warnings: Excessive amounts applied topically, especially to broken skin, may be absorbed and produce systemic toxic effects.
Administration: Topical.
Preparations: Powder, ointment and suppository.
Dose: As indicated by need.

BUTYN®, see Butacaine

C

CACAO BUTTER, see Theobroma
Oil

CADE OIL, see Juniper Tar

CAFFEINE
Stimulant. White powder, slightly soluble in water. Bitter taste. Found in effective amounts in coffee and tea.
Absorption: Well absorbed from G. I. tract.

Actions and Uses: Mild diuretic. Central stimulant action produces wakefulness, respiratory stimulation. Sometimes used together with analgesics for relief of headache.

Warnings: Overdosage may produce nervousness and wakefulness.

Administration: Oral.

Preparation: Powder and capsule.

Dose: 0.2 Gm.

CAFFEINE AND SODIUM BENZOATE

Stimulant. White, odorless powder, readily soluble in water. Bitter taste.

Actions and Uses: This mixture, containing about equal parts of caffeine and sodium benzoate, has all the properties of caffeine, but it is freely soluble and is therefore the preparation for parenteral injection.

Warnings: As for caffeine.

Administration: Oral, subcutaneous, intramuscular, intravenous.

Preparations: Ampule and powder, 0.25 Gm., 0.5 Gm. in 2 cc.

Dose: 0.5 Gm.

CALAMINE

Protective. Pink powder, tasteless, insoluble in water, but soluble in acids. Composed of zinc oxide with a small amount of ferric oxide.

Actions and Uses: Same as pure zinc oxide.

Administration: Topical.

Preparations: Liniment, and Lotion, 8% zinc oxide. Phenolated Lotion, 8% zinc oxide, 1% phenol.

Dose: Concentration, 8% zinc oxide.

CALCIFEROL, see Vitamin D

CALCIUM

Calcium is an element essential in the building and maintenance of bones. For this reason, large amounts are essential in growing children and pregnant females. The adult needs much smaller amounts. The utilization of calcium by bones is closely bound to vitamin D intake, and this vitamin must also be supplied in adequate amounts to prevent development of calcium disturbances. The parathyroid gland controls deposition of calcium in bones.

It is also a vital electrolyte in the blood, especially in relation to neuromuscular activity. In the case of low blood calcium levels, convulsions may develop.

Most important special purpose is its relationship to the toxic effects of lead. Calcium tends to keep lead in the bones, to prevent it from reaching high and toxic levels in the blood and to prevent the appearance of the symptoms of lead poisoning.

In large doses it may produce relaxation of muscle tone, and for that reason, it is sometimes given intravenously in cases of colic, especially lead colic.

Calcium chloride, Calcium chloride-Urea, Calcium gluconate, Calcium hydroxide, Calcium lactate, Calcuim levulinate, Calcium phosphate, Dicalcium phosphate.

CALCIUM AMINOSALICYLATE, see Para-Aminosalicylic Acid

CALCIUM BROMIDE

See Bromides.

CALCIUM CARBONATE—Precipitated Chalk

Antacid. Fine white powder, insoluble in water.

Absorption: Poor absorption from G. I. tract.

Actions and Uses: Gastric antacid with little tendency to "rebound" acidity. Used in diarrhea. Used as an ingredient of tooth powder.

Warnings: Liberates gas on contact with acid. Tends to produce constipation. Latter is overcome by mixing with magnesium carbonate.

Administration: Oral.

Preparations: Dentrifice, tablet, powder and combination with sodium bicarbonate in tablets.

Dose: 1 Gm.

CALCIUM CASEINATE—Aciban®

Calcium material used as antacid.

CALCIUM CHLORIDE

Source of calcium and urinary acidifier. White powder, soluble in water.

Absorption: Well absorbed from G. I. tract.

Actions and Uses: Provides calcium in states of calcium deficiency. An acid-forming diuretic. Used to relieve renal, biliary and lead colic and in lead poisoning.
Warnings: Said to increase the toxicity of digitalis, and to be used with caution in digitalized patients. Should not be used when kidneys are seriously injured. May cause G.I. disturbances. Inject slowly intravenously.
Administration: Oral, intravenous.
Preparations: Solution, for oral and parenteral use.
Dose: 0.5–1.0 Gm.

CALCIUM DISODIUM VERSENATE®, see Edathamil Calcium-Disodium

CALCIUM GLUCONATE
Source of calcium. White granules or powder, moderately soluble in water.
Absorption: Well absorbed from G. I. tract.
Actions and Uses: Much the same as calcium chloride as a source of calcium and often preferred to it because it causes no G. I. disturbances.
Warnings: As with calcium chloride.
Administrations: Oral, intravenous.
Preparations: Tablet and sterile solution.
Dose: 1–5 Gm.

CALCIUM GLYCEROPHOS-PHATE
Formerly used in neurasthenia, but there is no evidence that it is of any value.

CALCIUM HYDROXIDE—Slaked Lime
Antacid. White powder with bitter taste. Insoluble in water.
Absorption: Poorly absorbed from G. I. tract.
Actions and Uses: Antacid in gastric irritations and peptic ulcers.
Administration: Oral.
Preparations: Solution and lime water.
Dose: 15 cc. of a 3% solution.

CALCIUM HYPOPHOSPHITE
An ingredient of irrational "nerve tonics."

CALCIUM LACTATE
Source of calcium.

Actions and Uses: Same advantages over calcium chloride as the calcium gluconate.
Preparations: Tablet and solution.
Dose: 1 Gm.

CALCIUM LEVULINATE
Source of calcium.
A source of calcium which may be administered orally or intravenously. See Calcium.

CALCIUM MANDELATE
Urinary antiseptic.
Absorption: Well absorbed from G. I. tract.
Actions and Uses: Urinary antiseptic with the action of mandelic acid (which see). Also tends to acidify the urine.
Preparations: Tablet.
Dose: 3–4 Gm.

CALCIUM p-AMINOSALICYLATE
Antitubercular. Much the same as para-aminosalicylic acid, which see, with no proven advantages.

CALCIUM PHOSPHATE
Source of calcium. White powder, almost insoluble in water.
Absorption: Absorbed from G. I. tract.
Actions and Uses: Dietary supplement of calcium. Also may serve as a source of phosphorus.
Administration: Oral.
Preparations: Tablet.
Dose: 1 Gm.

CALOMEL, see Mercurous Chloride, Mild

CALSOL®, see Edathamil

CAMINOIDS®, see Aminopeptodrate

CAMOFORM®, see Biallylamicol

CAMOQUIN®, see Amodiaquin

CAMPHOR
Analeptic. White crystals, almost insoluble in water.
Actions and Uses: As a convulsant, may stimulate circulation and respiration. Formerly used for this purpose, but has given way to more effective drugs. Also of value as counterirritant. Mild antiseptic, and has local anesthetic action useful in treatment of itch.

CAMPHORATED TINCTURE OF OPIUM—Paregoric

Opium preparation. Brownish alcoholic solution with anise taste and odor.
Actions and Uses: Used mainly in treatment of diarrhea.
Warnings: Morphine content (0.4 mg. per cc.) is source of its effectiveness; continued use may lead to addiction.
Dose: 5 cc.

CANNABIS—Hashish, Marihuana

Not presently in use in medicine, but widely used illegally because of the unusual effects, mainly of a euphoric nature, produced by eating or smoking this drug. Highly addictive.

CANTHARIDES—Spanish Flies

Vesicant. Not used in modern medicine.
Warnings: May cause serious kidney damage if given internally.

CANTIL®, see Methyl-piperidyl-diphenylglycolate

CAPRYLIC ACID

Antifungal. Cream colored granules, usually the sodium salt, soluble in water; or the acid, an oily liquid.
Actions and Uses: Antifungal, much the same as propionic and undecylenic acid. Usually used in conjunction with other antifungal agents.

CAPRYLIC COMPOUND — Naprylate®

A mixture of sodium caprylate and zinc caprylate used as antifungal agent. See Caprylic Acid.

CAPSICUM—Cayenne Pepper

Carminative. Dark orange to brown powder with pungent taste and strong odor.
Actions and Uses: Rubefacient, carminative.
Warnings: May cause sneezing, local irritation.
Administration: Oral, topical.
Preparations: Ointment, oleoresin and tincture.
Dose: 60 mg.

CARAMIPHEN—Panparnit®, Toryn®

Anticholinergic, skeletal muscle relaxant, cough suppressant.

Actions and Uses: An anticholinergic material used, as others of the group, for the relaxation of skeletal muscle rigidity in the treatment of Parkinsonism. Also said to act directly on the cough center to depress the cough reflex and used, therefore, as a substitute for codeine in cough suppression but its value as such is yet to be established as being very great. Does not cause constipation.
Warnings: Considerably more trial is required before its claims for effectiveness are substantiated. The same danger of acute glaucoma is present here as in other atropine-like drugs. See Atropine.
Administration: Oral.
Preparations: Tablet, 10 mg. and Syrup.
Dose: 10 to 20 mg. every 4 hours if necessary.

CARBACHOL—Doryl®

Cholinergic. White or yellow crystals, soluble in water.
Absorption: Absorbed from G. I. tract.
Actions and Uses: Mimics stimulation of the vagus. Has prolonged effect. Used in intestinal ileus and urinary stasis.
Warnings: Overdosage may produce dangerous prolonged stimulation, vomiting, hypotension, bradycardia, asthmatic reaction. Do not use in intestinal obstruction.
Administration: Oral, subcutaneous.
Preparations: Tablet and sterile solution.
Dose: Oral, 2 mg. Subcutaneous, 0.25 mg.
Antidote: Atropine.

CARBACRYLAMINE RESINS— Carbo-Resin®

Exchange resin. A mixture containing potassium.
Actions and Uses: In relief of congestive heart failure as an adjuvant to treatment and a means of relieving the difficulties with the salt-poor diet. A sodium exchanger which removes sodium from food and the intestinal contents but provides enough potassium to prevent hypopotassemic reactions.
Warnings: Low-salt syndrome may develop insidiously, especially when used in conjunction with low-salt diet and other means of removing salt. Constipation and obstipation must be guarded against.

Administration: Oral.
Preparations: Powder.
Dose: 15 Gm. three times a day.

CARBAMIDE, see Urea

CARBAMIDE PEROXIDE—
Glycerite of Hydrogen Peroxide®
Antiseptic. A form of Hydrogen Peroxide, which see, which is said to be superior as a local antiseptic. Final evaluation will take some time. Used in 1.5 and 2.5% solutions.

CARBARSONE
Amebicide. White odorless powder, slightly acid taste, slightly soluble in water, contains arsenic.
Absorption: Absorbed from G.I. tract. Slowly eliminated.
Actions and Uses: For treatment of amebic dysentery.
Warnings: Do not use if patient has deep ulcerations in the colon, liver or kidney disease. There should be 10-day rest period between courses of treatment.
Administration: Oral, rectal.
Preparations: Vial, 2 Gm.; Capsule, 0.25 Gm., 50 mg.
Dose: Oral, 0.25 Gm. twice daily for 10 days, for adults. Rectal, 2 Gm. in 200 cc. water (containing sodium bicarbonate to facilitate solution) by retention enema, every other day for a total of 5 doses.
Antidote: Dimercaprol.

CARBASED®, see Acetylcarbromal

CARBAZOCHROME SALICYLATE
—Adrenosem Salicylate®,
Anaroxyl®
Hemostatic. Systemic hemostatic agent recommended for control of capillary bleeding due to increased capillary permeability. Does not affect blood clotting mechanism and is useless in massive hemorrhage. Status as a therapeutic agent remains to be established. Administered intramuscularly or orally in doses of from 1 to 5 mg., several times daily.

CARBETAPENTANE—Toclase®
Cough Suppressant. The citrate. Although not related to opium alkaloids, said to exert specific depressant action on cough center without dangers attaching to use of the latter. Much more experience is required to establish the importance and utility of this drug as an antitussive agent. Dermatitis has been reported following its use.
Preparations: Tablet, 25 mg. Syrup containing 7.5 mg. per teaspoonful and expectorant mixture of same concentration.
Dose: For adults 15 to 30 mg., several times daily.

CARBETHYL SALICYLATE—Salethyl Carbonate®
Non-addictive analgesic. No evidence of superiority over other salicylates. Available in 0.3 Gm. tablets.

CARBINOXAMINE—Clistin®
One of the large series of antihistamine drugs, which see.

CARBOL-FUCHSIN PAINT
—Carfusin®, Castellani's Paint
Fungicide. Deep violet solution; mixture of dye and other medicaments.
Actions and Uses: Suppresses epidermatophytosis and other superficial fungus infections of the skin.
Warnings: Do not use in acute lesions. Stains linen.
Administration: Topical.
Preparation: Solution contains boric acid, phenol, resorcinol, fuchsin, acetone, alcohol and water.
Dose: Apply as supplied.

CARBOLIC ACID, see Phenol

CARBOMYCIN—Magnamycin®
Antibiotic. A new antibiotic derived from *Streptomyces halstedii.*
Actions and Uses: Said to be effective against strains of staphylococci which are resistant to penicillin. Also effective in many other gram-positive and some rickettsial and large-virus infections. It is claimed that it is relatively nontoxic and that it does not disturb the normal bacterial flora of the intestine excessively.
Warnings: See antibiotics.
Administration: Oral.
Preparations: Tablet, 100 mg.
Dose: 100-300 mg. three times a day.

CARBON DIOXIDE
Respiratory stimulant. A colorless odorless gas, slightly soluble in water.
Absorption: Rapidly absorbed and eliminated from lungs.
Actions and Uses: Carbon dioxide is usually mixed with oxygen in anesthetic gases to stimulate respiration. Carbon dioxide snow (dry ice) is used as a refrigerant.
Warnings: Should not be administered in pure form. The "snow" should be used with care to avoid frostbite. Overinhalation of pure gas may induce anesthesia.
Administration: Inhalation (via mask) together with oxygen; topical.
Preparations: Pure gas, mixture with oxygen, 5-10%, in cylinder. Snow.
Dose: Amount necessary to produce stimulation of respiration, or to freeze.

CARBON TETRACHLORIDE
Vermifuge. Colorless liquid resembling chloroform in odor, with sweet taste. Decomposes slowly in light.
Absorption: Absorbed from G. I. tract. Inhaled fumes absorbed from lungs.
Actions and Uses: Widely used against hookworm and other intestinal parasites. Has narcotic and anesthetic properties.
Warnings: A highly toxic material, especially in alcoholic patients. May cause liver, kidney or even nerve injury. Fats, oil and alcohol should be avoided before administration. Largely replaced by more modern vermifuges.
Administration: Oral.
Preparations: Capsule, of 1-2.5 cc.
Dose: 2.5 cc. total at one time for an adult. Often preceded by a laxative. Given once, as a single dose; not repeated for at least 3 weeks.

CARBO-RESIN®, see Carbacrylamine Resins

CARBOWAX®, see Polyethylene Glycols

CARBOXYLIC RESINS—Natrinil®
Exchange Resin. Sodium removing type. See Exchange Resins.

CARBROMAL—Adalin®
Sedative. A white powder, slightly soluble in water.
Absorption: Absorbed from G.I. tract.
Actions and Uses: To induce sleep and relieve anxiety. Largely replaced for this purpose by more modern sedatives.
Warnings: Danger of habituation as with other sedative drugs.
Administration: Oral.
Preparations: Tablet.
Dose: 0.5 Gm.

CARDAMOM SEED
Carminative, Color. Brown to green powder.
Actions and Uses: As a flavor, carminative. Usually used in conjunction with other G. I. remedies.
Administration: Oral.
Preparations: Compound elixir, oil, spirit, compound tincture.
Dose: Variable, depending upon purpose.

CARDIAC DEPRESSANTS—
Procaine amide, Quinidine.

CARDIAC STIMULANTS
Adrenergics, digitalis materials, Methylamino-hydroxy-methylheptane.

CARFUSIN®, see Carbol-Fuchsin Paint

CARONAMIDE—Staticin®
Renal blocking agent. Formerly used to prolong penicillin action, little used at present. Available in 0.5 Gm. tablets.

CAROTENE—Pro-Vitamin A
Carotene is converted in the body into Vitamin A and may, therefore, be used instead of it. See Oleovitamin A.

CASCARA SAGRADA
Cathartic. Dried bark, powdered. Yellow color. Bitter taste.
Actions and Uses: Mild laxative, acting mainly on the colon.
Warnings: Like all laxatives, tends to induce dependence when used regularly.
Administration: Oral.
Preparations: Tablet, fluidextract and aromatic fluidextract.
Dose: Equivalent of 0.3 Gm. of the extract. Best result obtained if given in small doses after meals.

CASSIA PODS—Senokot®
Cathartic. Available in granules and tablets.

CASTELLANI'S PAINT, see
Carbol-Fuchsin Paint

CASTILE SOAP, see Soap, Hard

CASTOR OIL
Cathartic. Yellow or colorless viscid oil. Usually has nauseating taste.
Actions and Uses: Prompt and effective cathartic with tendency to induce griping.
Warnings: Likely to be followed by constipation and like all cathartics, its continued use is apt to induce dependence.
Administration: Oral.
Preparations: Oil. Capsule, aromatic oil. Ointment, castor oil and bismuth subnitrate, castor oil and zinc oxide.
Dose: Usually 15 cc.

CATHARTICS—Laxatives, Purgatives
Agar, Aloe, Aloin, Bile salts, Cascara sagrada, Cassia pods, Castor oil, Dioctyl sodium sulfosuccinate, Dihydroxyanthraquinone, Jalap, Magnesia magma, Magnesium hydroxide, Magnesium sulfate (Epsom salts), Mercurous chloride, mild, Methylcellulose, Petrolatum, Phenolphthalein, Plantago (Psyllium), Rhubarb, Senna, Sodium phosphate, Sodium sulfate.

CATHOMYCIN®, see Novobiocin

CAUSTIC SODA, see Sodium Hydroxide

CAUSTICS
Acetpyrogall, Bichloracetic acid, Chromium trioxide, Mercury bichloride, Monochloracetic acid, Nitric acid, Phenol, Silver nitrate, Sodium hydroxide, Trichloracetic acid.

CAYENNE PEPPER, see Capsicum

CEBIONE®, see Ascorbic Acid

CEDILANID®, see Lanatoside C

CEDILANID-D®, see Deslanoside

CEEPRYN®, see Cetyl Pyridinium

CELLOTHYL®, see Methylcellulose

CELLULOSE, OXIDIZED—Hemo-Pak®

Hemostatic. Gauze or cotton, white. Insoluble in water.
Actions and Uses: Hemostatic, which is absorbed when buried in tissues. Used in surgery.
Preparations: Absorbable pad and packing strips.

CENTRINE®, see Aminopentamide

CER-O-CILLIN®, see Potassium Penicillin O

CETYL PYRIDINIUM—Ceepryn®
Antiseptic. White powder soluble in water, the chloride.
Actions and Uses: A detergent type of antiseptic used in preparation of skin for operation, topical application to mucous membranes and for sterilization of instruments.
Warnings: Inactivated by soap; not effective against spores.
Administration: Topical.
Preparations: Solution, 10% and 0.1%. Tincture, 1:200 and 1:500, may be tinted.
Dose: Concentration used depends on tissue and indications.

CEVEX®, see Ascorbic Acid

CEVITAMIC ACID, see Ascorbic Acid

CHALK, PRECIPITATED, see Calcium Carbonate

CHARCOAL, ACTIVATED
Adsorbent. Charcoal, fine black powder.
Actions and Uses: Adsorbent of gases, used internally for this purpose, but of doubtful value.
Administration: Oral.
Preparations: Tablet and powder.
Dose: 1 Gm.

CHAULMOOGRA OIL
Actions and Uses: Replaced by more effective modern antibiotics and chemotherapeutic agents in the treatment of tuberculosis.

CHENOPODIUM OIL—Wormseed Oil
Vermifuge. Yellow oil with unpleasant odor and bitter burning taste.
Actions and Uses: For treatment of

roundworms and hookworms. Largely replaced by less toxic drugs.
Warnings: Contraindicated in liver, heart and kidney disease. Toxic reactions, which may be delayed, consist of ringing in the ears, deafness, impaired vision, headache, nausea, vomiting, respiratory depression, convulsions, coma, death.
Administration: Oral.
Preparations: Capsule.
Dose: 0.2 cc. every 1-2 hours for a maximum of 5 doses. Should be followed by saline cathartic.

CHERRY, WILD, see Wild Cherry Syrup

CHINIOFON—Anayodin®, Yatren®
Amebicide. Yellow powder with bitter taste, moderately soluble in water. Contains about 27% iodine. Effervesces when mixed with water. Deteriorates in light.
Actions and Uses: Used in treatment of amebic dysentery.
Warnings: High iodine content necessitates special caution in patients with thyroid disease. Also special danger in patients with liver disease.
Administration: Oral, rectal.
Preparations: Tablet 0.25 Gm., enteric coated. Vial, 3 Gm.
Dose: Oral, 0.5-1.0 Gm. 3 times daily for 7-14 days. Rectal, 3 Gm. in 300 cc. water by retention enema. When both oral and rectal routes are used simultaneously, dose given by each route should be halved. May also be used simultaneously with emetine.

CHLORAL HYDRATE—Notec®, Somnos®
Sedative. White aromatic crystals with bitter taste. Very soluble in water.
Absorption: Well absorbed from G. I. tract and relatively rapidly eliminated.
Actions and Uses: Relatively potent hypnotic and sedative, to alleviate nervousness and insomnia.
Warnings: Continued use may induce habituation. Untoward effects may result from toxic doses, especially in cardiac patients and those with liver disease. Dis-

agreeable to take in solution orally because of taste.
Administration: Oral.
Preparations: Capsule and solution, flavored with peppermint water.
Dose: 0.6 Gm.

CHLORAMBUCIL—Leukeran®
Antileukemic. Nitrogen mustard available in 2 mg. tablets.

CHLORAMPHENICOL—Chloromycetin®
Antibiotic. White crystals with bitter taste, slightly soluble in water.
Absorption: From G. I. tract.
Actions and Uses: A so-called "wide spectrum" antibiotic with effectiveness against many gram-negative organisms, rickettsial bodies, atypical pneumonia, typhoid and others. It is used only when other antibiotics are not effective.
Warnings: Anemia and fatal granulocytopenia have been reported; in addition, the usual warnings against the indiscriminate use of antibiotics should be observed.
Administration: Oral.
Preparations: Capsule, 250 mg., 50 mg.
Dose: 3-5 Gm. daily, depending on the condition, in 4 doses per 24 hour period.

CHLORCYCLIZINE—Di-Paralene®, Perazil®
An antihistaminic, which see.

CHLORESIUM®, see Chlorophyll

CHLORETONE®, see Chlorobutanol

CHLORINE
Many chlorine compounds exert a germicidal effect when they liberate free chlorine. This action has long been used in medicine for local antiseptic action on the skin and in wounds, and for the disinfection of drapes, instruments, clothing and contaminated objects. Dakin's solution, Labarraque's solution and Javelle water are well known examples of these. The disadvantage of these solutions is their instability; in general, they must be quite fresh to be effective. There are, however, more modern drugs which are somewhat more stable in solution.

Chloramine-T, Chlorazodin, Dichloramine-T, Halazone, Sodium Hypochlorite, Succinchlorimide.

CHLORIODIZED OIL—
Iodochlorol®

X-ray medium. Yellow oil, containing about 37% iodine. Deteriorates in light.
Actions and Uses: Used for x-ray visualization of bronchial tree, female genital tract and spinal canal.
Administration: Instillation into area for visualization.
Preparations: Liquid.
Dose: Amount required for the particular condition.

CHLORISONDAMINE—Ecolid®
Hypotensive. A new ganglionic blockader whose real uses and dangers remain to be established. Dosage of the order of 25 mg. starting once daily and gradually increased to three times a day.

CHLORMERODRIN—Neohydrin®
Mercurial diuretic.
Actions and Uses: Oral diuretic for use in the control of edema in all types of cardiac disease, including hypertension.
Administration: Oral.
Preparations: Tablet, 18.3 mg. of active drug.
Warnings: Gastro-intestinal irritation is common. See Mercury.
Dose: 1 tablet or more daily.
Antidote: Dimercaprol.

CHLOROAZODIN—
Azochloramid®

Antiseptic. Yellow needles or flakes with slight odor like chlorine. Decomposes on exposure to light. Slightly soluble in water. Decomposes on contact with metals.
Actions and Uses: To disinfect mucous membranes of vagina, rectum and colon. Of doubtful value.
Warnings: Do not use in concentrated solution.
Administration: Topical.
Preparations: Solution.
Dose: Concentration, 1:1500 to 1:3000.

CHLOROBUTANOL—
Chloretone®, Clortran®

Hypnotic and preservative. White crystals with camphor-like odor. Moderately soluble in water.
Actions and Uses: Hypnotic and general anesthetic. It also has a moderate antiseptic action, and it is for this action that it is now used more than for any other; added to solutions as a preservative.
Warnings: Danger of habituation same as with other sedative drugs.
Administration: Oral.
Preparations: Tablet.
Dose: 0.6 Gm.

CHLOROFORM
Anesthetic, rubefacient and solvent. Colorless heavy fluid with sweetish taste and characteristic odor.
Absorption: Absorbed from G. I. tract and vapors are absorbed from the lungs. Deteriorates in light.
Actions and Uses: An effective general anesthetic for which purpose it has been entirely discarded because of dangers of cardiac depression. Now used as local irritant in liniments.
Warnings: Dangerous as an anesthetic. May cause blistering from local application.
Administration: Topical.
Preparations: Liniment, containing about 30% chloroform.
Dose: As indicated by effect locally.

CHLOROGUANIDE—Guanatol®,
Paludrine®, Proguanil

Antimalarial. Colorless crystals with bitter taste, usually the hydrochloride. Darkens on exposure to light. Moderately soluble in water.
Actions and Uses: Prophylaxis, suppression and treatment of malignant tertian and certain forms of benign tertian malaria. Notable for its lack of toxicity to man.
Administration: Oral.
Preparations: Tablet, 25, 50, 100, 300 mg.
Dose: Suppression, 0.3 Gm. weekly. Prophylaxis, 0.1 Gm. twice weekly. Treatment, 0.1 Gm. three times daily for 10 days.

CHLOROMYCETIN®, see Chloramphenicol

CHLOROPHENOTHANE—DDT
Antiparasitic. White crystals, insoluble in water.
Absorption: Slowly absorbed from G. l. tract.
Actions and Uses: Used to eradicate bed bugs, lice, flies, mosquitoes, and many other insects.
Warnings: Toxic to humans.
Administration: Spray, dust.
Preparations: Liquid for spray and powder for dusting. Combinations with other insecticides.
Dose: Concentration usually 5–10% in sprays; 1% in medicaments.

CHLOROPHYLL—Chloresium®
Deodorizing agent. Water soluble chlorophyll containing substance, frequently in the form of sodium or potassium salts.
Actions and Uses: Used for deodorization, normal tissue repair and relief of itching in wounds, ulcers, burns, dermatoses. Conclusive evidence is lacking that derivatives stimulate granulation or that it has any merit as a deodorant.
Warnings: There is no evidence of curative or even deodorant value.
Administration: Oral, topical.
Preparations: Tablet. Ointment, 0.5%. Solution, 0.2%. Dentifrice.
Dose: Varies as indicated.

CHLOROPROCAINE—Nescaine®
Local anesthetic. Advantages over procaine, which it closely resembles, remain to be established. Available in 2 and 3% solutions.

CHLOROPROCAINE PENICIL-LIN O—Depo-Cer-O-Cillin Chloroprocaine®
Another form of penicillin said to be less allergenic than Penicillin G. See Penicillin.

CHLOROQUINE—Aralen®
Antimalarial. White powder, with a bitter taste, usually the phosphate. Discolors on exposure to light. Very soluble in water.
Actions and Uses: Used to suppress and treat certain forms of malaria and extraintestinal amebiasis.
Warnings: Overdosage may cause blurring of vision, pruritus, headache, G. I. upsets. In suppressive dosage, serious effects are rare and tend to disappear as soon as the drug is discontinued.
Administration: Oral.
Preparations: Tablet, 0.25 Gm.
Dose: Suppression, 0.5 Gm. weekly. Treatment, 1 Gm. and 0.5 Gm. in 6 hours, then 0.5 Gm. daily for 2 days. Amebiasis, 1 Gm. daily in divided doses for 2 days followed by 0.25 Gm. twice daily for 2-3 weeks.

CHLOROTHEN—Tagathen®
An antihistaminic, which see.

CHLOROTRIANISENE—TACE®
A synthetic estrogen. See Estrogens.

CHLORPROMAZINE—Thorazine®
Antiemetic. The hydrochloride.
Actions and Uses: Basically an antihistaminic drug which is claimed to have an exceptionally well developed antinauseant and antiemetic action and useful in virtually all types of nausea and vomiting, including radiation sickness and carcinoma. Exerts strong sedative action for which it may be used in excitement. Also said to potentiate addictive analgesics and, therefore, to reduce the amount of these drugs required for the relief of pain. Because of central depressant action is now widely used for relief of anxiety and excitement, especially in psychotic patients. At present this is, perhaps, its greatest use.
Warnings: This is an exceedingly new drug and the extent of its toxic potential has not yet been determined. Serious accidents following its use have already been reported; jaundice is not rare. Its intense sedative action constitutes one of its great hazards in its use in ambulant patients. With continued use bone marrow depression has been observed; regular blood counts are, therefore, indicated in such cases.
Administration: Oral and parenteral.

Preparations: Tablets, 10 and 25 mg. Ampules, 2 cc. (25 mg. per cc.).
Dose: 10 to 50 mg. as indicated.

CHLORPHENIRAMINE—Chlortrimeton®, Teldrin®
An antihistaminic, which see.

CHLORQUINALDOL—Sterosan®
Antiseptic, antifungal. Used mainly in treatment of skin infections. Administered topically, usually in a 3% ointment or cream.

CHLORTETRACYCLINE—Aureomycin®
Antibiotic. A yellowish powder, the hydrochloride, obtained from *Streptomyces aureofaciens.* Bitter taste. Very slightly soluble in water.
Absorption: Well absorbed from G. I. tract.
Actions and Uses: An effective agent in many rickettsial diseases, staphylococcic and pneumococcic infections, atypical pneumonia, some streptococcic infections, some infections of the urinary tract, brucellosis and in some viral infections.
Warnings: G. I. upsets and diarrhea are common. Prolonged use may lead to skin eruptions around mouth and anus; may result in monilia infections.
Administration: Oral, parenteral.
Preparations: Capsule, 50 mg., 250 mg. Vial, parenteral preparation to be dissolved just before using. Ophthalmic ointment, solution.
Dose: 0.5 Gm. every 6 hours.

CHLOR-TRIMETON®, see Chlorpheniramine

CHOLEDYL®, see Oxtriphylline

CHOLERETICS
Bile salts, Dehydrocholic acid, Lecithin compound, Ox bile extract.

CHOLINE DIHYDROGEN CITRATE—Chothyn®
Nutritional. A fatty material.
Actions and Uses: Lipotropic agent for treatment of cirrhosis of liver and other hepatic disease.
Warnings: Not of proven value and should not replace other aspects of die-

tary therapy in hepatic disease. Dose should not exceed 6 Gm. daily.
Administration: Oral.
Preparations: Capsule, 1.0 Gm., 0.5 Gm. Tablet, 0.5 Gm., 0.65 Gm. Syrup, 1 Gm. in 4 cc.
Dose: 1-2 Gm. 2-3 times daily.

CHOLINE GLUCONATE
Lipotropic. Same properties as Choline Dihydrogen Citrate, which see.

CHOLINERGICS
Ambenomium, Benzpyrinium, Bethanechol, Carbachol, Furtrethonium, Isoflurophate, Methacholine, Neostigmine, Physostigmine, Pilocarpine, Pyridostigmin.

CHOLINE THEOPHYLLINATE, see Oxtriphylline

CHOLOGRAFIN®, see Iodipamide

CHONDODENDRON TOMENTOSUM EXTRACT—Intocostrin®
Anticonvulsant.
An aqueous extract of crude curare and exerting the actions of curare. See tubocurarine.

CHOTHYN®, see Choline Dihydrogen Citrate

CHROMIC ACID, see Chromium Trioxide

CHROMIUM TRIOXIDE—Chromic Acid
Caustic. Purplish crystals, soluble in water.
Actions and Uses: A powerful caustic whose action is difficult to control. Used for removal of warts and other foreign growth. In dilute solutions (5%), an astringent wash; in somewhat stronger concentrations (up to 10%), used in treatment of Vincent's Angina.
Warnings: Extremely caustic and may cause deep ulcerations in concentrated form. Explosive when mixed with organic matter in concentrated state.
Administration: Topical.
Preparations: Solution.
Dose: Concentration as indicated.

CHRYSAROBIN
Parasiticide. Brown to orange powder, irritant to mucous membranes. Has keratolytic action.

Actions and Uses: Antiparasitic and skin irritant used in treatment of psoriasis, ringworm, chronic eczema and other skin conditions.
Warnings: May cause skin destruction, permanent staining of linen and skin. Benzene will remove stains to linens. Absorption from the skin may cause kidney damage.
Administration: Topical.
Preparations: Ointment.
Dose: Concentration, 2-10%.

CHYMAR®, see Chymotrypsin

CHYMOTRYPSIN—Chymar®, Enzeon®
Proteolytic enzyme. Recommended for inflammatory conditions. Value to be established and, until then, to be questioned. Administered intramuscularly.

CIGNOLIN®, see Anthralin

CINAPHYL®, see Theophylline Sodium Glycinate

CINCHONA
Antimalarial.
Cinchona is obtained from bark of the cinchona tree and contains several alkaloidal materials which are effective in treatment of malaria and constitute the oldest specific drugs in common use. Chief of these drugs is quinine which is discussed elsewhere. Quinidine is another of these alkaloids which also has an important cardiac action. There are also cinchonidine and cinchonine, which are almost as effective as quinine and quinidine as antimalarial agents. They are rarely used, mainly because the bark does not contain as much of these as the other alkaloids; the statement that they are more difficult to use is not supported by good evidence. The cinchona alkaloids also exert analgesic and anti-pyretic actions.
Finally, the crude bark, or simple extracts of the bark containing all the alkaloids, have been used effectively in the treatment of malaria. Totaquine is one of these. It has the advantage of being considerably cheaper because much effort has not been expended in the process of purification. To a large extent, however, cinchona has been supplanted by the more effective and less toxic newer antimalarial agents. In general, the undesirable effects of all the cinchona alkaloids are about the same.

CINCHOPHEN—Atophan®
Analgesic and antipyretic. Small white crystals with slightly bitter taste. Insoluble in water.
Actions and Uses: Effective as a general analgesic and antipyretic, much as aspirin.
Warnings: Serious liver damage may follow its use in hypersensitive patients.
Administration: Oral.
Preparations: Tablet.
Dose: 0.3-0.5 Gm.

CINNAMON
Carminative. Yellowish or reddish brown powder with spicy taste.
Actions and Uses: Carminative or aromatic, for flavoring.
Preparations: Powder, oil, spirit, tincture, water.

CITRATE OF MAGNESIA, see Magnesium Citrate

CLISTIN®, see Carbinoxamine

CLOPANE®, see Cyclopentamine

CLORARSEN®—Dichlorophenarsine, see Arsenic

CLORTRAN®, see Chlorobutanol

CLOVE OIL
Counterirritant and local anesthetic. Colorless or pale yellow liquid, darkening with age. Has a characteristic taste of cloves.
Actions and Uses: Counterirritant; local anesthetic for cavities in teeth.
Warnings: Store in cool, dark place.
Administration: Topical, oral.
Preparations: Oil.
Dose: 0.1-0.4 cc.

COAL TAR—Crude Coal Tar
Antiseptic.
Black, thick liquid with characteristic odor and burning taste.

Actions and Uses: Antiseptic and irritant for treatment of skin diseases.
Warnings: May cause severe irritation if used for long periods of time.
Administration: Topical.
Preparations: Cream, ointment, solution.
Dose: Concentration, 1-5%.

COCAINE
Local anesthetic. White crystals or powder. Salts are soluble in water.
Absorption: Rapidly absorbed from mucous membranes, cuts and abrasions in mucous membranes and from G. I. tract.
Actions and Uses: A potent local anesthetic, which is especially outstanding because of its action on mucous membranes. It is also a powerful central nervous system stimulant and produces effects which lead to addiction.
Warnings: The dangers from rapid absorption are great and special care should be taken not to apply the drug to mucous membranes with cuts or erosions. Wherever possible, a safer substitute should be used. Frequent use may lead to addiction. Under control of federal narcotic laws.
Administration: Topical.
Preparations: Solution, ointment, tablet and capsule.
Dose: Concentration, 0.5–10% for local anesthesia.
Antidote: Barbiturate.

COCOA BUTTER, see Theobroma Oil

CODEINE
Addictive analgesic. White crystals. Salts are soluble in water. Extremely bitter.
Absorption: Well absorbed from G. I. tract. Excreted in several hours.
Actions and Uses: An effective analgesic preferred to morphine because of decreased addiction potential. Is made from morphine and closely resembles it in all its actions, except that it is less potent and produces less euphoria. Suppresses cough reflex and is, therefore, used in many cough remedies. Constipating.
Warnings: Danger of addiction from continued use is more likely than is generally recognized. Induces obstinate constipation. Under the control of federal and state narcotic laws.
Administration: Oral, subcutaneous.
Preparations: Tablet, oral and parenteral solution. Cough mixtures (codeine and ipecac, codeine and terpin hydrate, codeine and wild cherry).
Dose: Suppression of cough, 8 mg. Analgesic, 15—65 mg.
Antidote: Nalorphine.

COD LIVER OIL
Vitamin. An oily liquid with a characteristic fishy odor and taste.
Actions and Uses: For prevention and treatment of vitamin A and D deficiencies. In many instances, this has been replaced by concentrates and purer forms of these vitamins. The latter forms are now relatively inexpensive, and much simpler to administer. The oil has, in addition to its other properties, a high caloric value as a food.
Administration: Oral, topical.
Preparations: Oil, emulsion, emulsion with malt and flavors, capsule, concentrate, tablet, ointment (used locally for certain skin eruptions.)
Dose: 8 cc. daily for prevention of ricketts in children.

COGENTIN®, see Benztropine

COLACE®, see Dioctyl Sodium Sulfosuccinate

COLCHICINE
Analgesic. Yellow scales or powder.
Absorption: Well absorbed from G. I. tract.
Actions and Uses: Analgesic for treatment of gout. Also has a marked irritant action on the intestinal tract and kidneys.
Warnings: A relatively dangerous drug. May produce diarrhea, watery stools, enteritis, nephritis and collapse. Effective doses generally produce diarrhea, and this may be taken as a sign to stop the medication, or at least, to decrease the dose.
Administration: Oral.
Preparations: Tablet and tincture.
Dose: 0.5 mg. of the pure alkaloid.

COLLODION, FLEXIBLE
Vehicle and protective. A pale yellow viscid fluid with ethereal odor, which evaporates quickly, leaving a thick skin-like film.
Actions and Uses: Used for application of local medications and as a protective.
Warnings: Volatile and inflammable. Keep tightly stoppered and away from open flame.

COLPROSTERONE®, see Progesterone

COMBIOTIC®
Antibiotic. A mixture of Procaine Penicillin and Dihydrostreptomycin.

COMPENAMINE®, see Ephenamine Penicillin G

COMPAZINE®, see Prochlorperazine

COMPOCILLIN®, see Hydrabamine Penicillin G

CONESTRON®, see Estrogenic Substances, Conjugated

CONGO RED
Diagnostic. Dark red powder, moderately soluble in water.
Actions and Uses: Disappears with unusual rapidity from the blood stream in cases of amyloid disease. Used in a test based on this phenomenon.
Warnings: Excessive dose, or too rapid injection, may cause intravascular clotting.
Administration: Intravenous.
Preparations: Ampule, 10 or 20 cc. of 1% solution.
Dose: 10–20 cc. of 1% solution.

COPARAFFINATE—Iso-Par®
Antifungal agent.

COPSAMINE®, see Pyrilamine

CORAMINE®, see Nikethamide

CORLUTONE®, see Progesterone

CORN OIL—Maize Oil
Edible oil. Clear, light yellow oil with faint taste and odor.
Actions and Uses: As a vehicle or food. Said to have special values in certain forms of eczema because of a high content of unsaturated fatty acids.

Warnings: Excessive amounts may cause diarrhea. Stopper tightly and store in cool place to prevent rancidity.

CORTATE®, see Desoxycorticosterone

CORTEF®, see Hydrocortisone

CORTICOTROPIN — Adrenocorticotropic Hormone, ACTH, Acthar®, Acthar Gel®, Cortrophin®, Depo-ACTH®, Solacthyl®
Hormone. Lyophilized powder or gel, soluble in water. Standardized in Units, each equal to 1 mg. Obtained from anterior pituitary glands of cattle.
Actions and Uses: Much the same as cortisone; produces its effects on the adrenal cortex, which in turn exerts cortisone-like action. Used in mesenchymal diseases in general.
Warnings: Much as with cortisone. Local reactions common. May induce diabetes, interfere with the control of congestive heart failure, cause psychic disturbances, skin eruptions, etc.
Administration: Intramuscular, intravenous.
Preparations: Ampule, powder to be dissolved before using—10, 15, 25, 40 Units. Acthar Gel, multiple dose vials—20, 40 Units. Sterile syringes—20, 40 Units. Zinc salt.
Dose: Variable, depending on condition. 10-25 Units every 6 hours. Large doses less frequently with repository (gel) form. Zinc salt requires smaller dosage because of prolonged activity.

CORTICOTROPHIN-ZINC, see Corticotropin

CORTISONE—Cortogen®, Cortone®
Hormone. Acetate, white odorless powder, insoluble in water.
Absorption: Absorbed from G. I. tract.
Actions and Uses: Much like ACTH. Used in treatment of arthritis, rheumatic fever, lupus erythematosis and other collagen diseases. Does not cure. Also for acute allergic reactions, gout, Bell's palsy and other diseases.
Warnings: Dangerous, except in the hands

of the experienced. May produce diabetes, psychoses, neurologic symptoms,
hypopotassemia, edema. Interferes with
control of congestive heart failure and
the healing of wounds. Gastric ulcers
have been reported after long continued
use.
Administration: Oral, intramuscular.
Preparations: Tablet, 5 mg., 25 mg. Vial,
500 mg., to be dissolved, 25 mg. per cc.
Dose: 300 mg. first day, 100 mg. daily
thereafter. Divided into 4 doses daily.

CORTOGEN®, see Cortisone

CORTONE®, see Cortisone

CORTRIL®, see Hydrocortisone

CORTROPHIN®, see Corticotropin

COTINAZIN®, see Isoniazid

COTTONSEED OIL
Edible oil. Pale yellow, or colorless oil.
Nearly odorless and tasteless.
Actions and Uses: Vehicle and food.
Large doses have laxative action. Often
used in enemas, especially to relieve
fecal impactions. May be substituted for
other forms of fat in allergic patients.
Warnings: Stopper tightly and store in
cool place to prevent rancidity.

COUGH SUPPRESSANTS
Caramiphen, Carbetapentamine, Codeine,
Dextromethorphan, Dihydrocodeinone,
Morphine.

COUMADIN®, see Warfarin

COUMARIN DERIVATIVES
Bishydroxycoumarin (Dicumarol®) is the
first of a now growing series of related
(and some unrelated) drugs which are
being introduced as anticoagulants. The
disadvantage of the Dicumarol® is the
delay before its effect and the variability
of its effect on the blood-clotting mechanism. One, Warfarin, is used as a
rodenticide because of this type of action
in rats and mice. The newer derivatives
are usually stated to have advantages
over the Dicumarol® in this respect. In
most instances these drugs are far too
new to state whether this is actually
the case.
Acenocoumarin, Bishydroxycoumarin, Cyclocumarol, Ethylbiscoumarate, Warfarin.

COVICONE®, see Dimethicone

CR⁵¹, see Radio-Chromate Sodium

CREAMALIN®, see Aluminum Hydroxide Gel

CRESOL
Antiseptic. Colorless to brownish liquid
with characteristic odor, becoming darker
on age and exposure to light. Forms a
cloudy solution when mixed with water.
Actions and Uses: A potent disinfectant,
approximately 4 times as potent as phenol and perhaps no more toxic. Used for
disinfection of instruments, drapes, clothing, rooms, etc.
Warnings: Highly irritant to skin. Highly
toxic orally. Should any splash on eye,
wash promptly with water of solution of
sodium bicarbonate.
Preparations: Saponated solution of Cresol, 50% cresol.
Dose: Concentrations vary as indicated
by need.

CROTAMITON—Eurax®
Antipruritic.
Actions and uses: Claimed to relieve
intense itching of a wide variety of
causes.
Warnings: Do not use in acute, severe
dermatitis, especially when skin is
abraded.
Administration: Topical.
Preparations: Cream, 10%.

CRUDE OIL TAR, see Coal Tar

CRYPTENAMINE—Unitensin®
Hypotensive. Veratrum preparation, which
see.
Available in vials, 2 mg. per cc. Dosage
depends on condition and reaction of
patient who should be carefully watched
during treatment.

**CRYSTAL VIOLET, see Methyl-
rosaniline**

CRYSTICILLIN®, see Penicillin G

CRYSTODIGIN®, see Digitoxin

CRYSTOSERPINE®, see Reserpine

CUMERTILIN®, see Mercumatilin

CUMOPYRAN®, see Cyclocumarol

CUPRIC SULPHATE—Blue Vitriol
Astringent. Blue crystals or powder, soluble in water.
Actions and Uses: Astringent when applied locally. By mouth, it is a G. I. irritant and emetic. Effective antidote in phosphorus poisoning. Extremely toxic. Antiseptic action in water. Omitted from most hospital formularies.
Warnings: May cause serious and fatal G. I. and kidney damage. Never indicated in modern medicine for internal use, except perhaps in the case of phosphorus poisoning. Use as an emetic may be dangerous.
Administration: Topical, oral (in phosphorus poisoning).
Dose: A single dose of 0.3 Gm. in solution in phosphorus poisoning, not to be repeated. Topical, concentration varies depending upon use.

CURARE, see Tubocurarine

CYANOCOBALAMIN, see Vitamin B$_{12}$

CYCLAINE®, see Hexylcaine

CYCLAMATE—Sucaryl®
Sugar substitute. The sodium salt, white, soluble, sweet crystals. 30 times as sweet as cane sugar.
Actions and Uses: Noncaloric sugar substitute where sugar-intake is restricted.
Warnings: Sodium content must be considered if sodium is also restricted.
Preparations: 15% solution, 0.12 Gm. tablets.
Dose: Daily dose should not exceed 1.5 Gm.

CYCLIZINE—Marezine®
One of the large group of antihistaminic drugs; this one, however, is said to have special value in the treatment and prevention of nausea and vomiting and motion sickness. See Antihistaminics.

CYCLOBARBITAL—Phanodorn®
One of the rapid acting barbiturates, which see.

CYCLOCUMAROL—Cumopyran®
Anticoagulant. Another coumarin derivative with the properties and dangers of the group.

Dosage of the same order as Bishydroxycoumarin (Dicumarol®). See Coumarin Derivatives.

CYCLOGYL®, see Cyclopentolate

CYCLOMETHYCAINE—
Surfacaine®
Topical anesthetic. New drug, relative merits and dangers remain to be established by clinical trial.

CYCLOPENTAMINE—Clopane®
One of the large series of adrenergic drugs, which see. Used especially for nasal decongestant action.

CYCLOPENTOLATE—Cyclogyl®
One of the long list of anticholinergic drugs with much the same actions and dangers as atropine, which see.

CYCLOPROPANE
General anesthetic. Colorless gas with characteristic odor, pungent taste. Inflammable.
Actions and Uses: Used for surgical anesthesia by inhalation. Tends to produce cardiac arrhythmias. Less irritating than ether.
Warnings: Usually contraindicated in cases complicated by cardiac disease, especially those with a tendency to arrhythmias. Not to be used by those without experience with this gas. Extreme precautions must be taken to prevent explosion in the operating room.
Administration: Inhalation (with oxygen).
Preparations: Cylinders containing pure cyclopropane.
Dose: As indicated by state of patient.

CYCLOSERINE—Seromycin®
Antibiotic. New antibiotic obtained from *Streptomyces orchidaceus* which is effective in common urinary tract infections and in tuberculosis. Advantages over Streptomycin remain to be established. Convulsions have been reported following its use.

CYCRIMINE—Pagitane®
Muscle relaxant, anticholinergic. White bitter powder.
Actions and Uses: Muscle relaxant with anticholinergic properties. Used in the

relief of the muscle rigidity of Parkinsonism.
Warnings: In common with all anticholinergic drugs may induce acute glaucoma in sensitive patients.
Administration: Oral.
Preparations: Tablets, 1.25 and 2.5 mg.
Dose: 1.25 mg. three times daily.

CYTELLIN®, see Sitosterols

CYTOMEL®, see Liothyronine

D

DACTIL®, see Piperidolate

DAKIN'S SOLUTION, see Sodium Hypochlorite

d-AMFETASUL®, see Dextro Amphetamine

DANILONE®, see Phenindione

DARAPRIM®, see Pyrimethamine

DARROW'S SOLUTION—see Potassic Saline

DARVON®, see Dextro Propoxyphene

DASEROL®, see Mephenesin

DDT, see Chlorophenothane

DECAMETHONIUM—Syncurine®
Skeletal muscle relaxant. Used in much the same way as curare-like drugs for anesthesia and electro-shock therapy. Further examination necessary for final evaluation. Dosage of the order of 0.5 to 3.0 mg. intravenously.

DECAPRYN®, see Doxylamine

DECHOLIN®, see Dehydrocholic Acid

DECONGESTANTS (nasal), see Adrenergics

DEHYDROCHOLIC ACID— Decholin®
Choleretic and diagnostic.
Actions and Uses: Stimulates the flow of bile and hastens filling of gall-bladder, not its emptying. Used for a test of circulation time which is based on the fact that after injection into a vein, the material circulates through the body and reaches the taste buds of the tongue, where it produces a bitter taste. Has a weak diuretic action.
Warnings: Contraindicated in cases of complete biliary obstruction. May induce asthmatic attacks in patients with asthma. Use carefully in patients with hepatitis.
Administration: Oral.
Preparations: Tablets, 0.25 Gm.
Dose: 1-2 tablets, three times a day.

DELALUTIN®, see Hydroxyprogesterone

DELATESTRYL®, see Testosterone Enanthate

DELESTROGEN®, see Estradiol Valerate

DELTA-CORTEF®, see Prednisolone

DELTASONE®, see Prednisone

DELTRA®, see Prednisone

DELVINAL®, see Vinbarbital

DELYSID®, see Lysergic Acid Diethylamide

DEMEROL®, see Meperidine

DEPO-ACTH®, see Corticotropin

DEPO-CER-O-CILLIN CHLOROPROCAINE®, see Chloroprocaine Penicillin O

DEPROPANEX®
Vasodilator. A defatted, water-soluble, insulin-free, deproteinated extract of pancreatic tissue.
Actions and Uses: Said to induce peripheral arterial vasodilation and used, therefore, in arteriosclerotic disease of the extremities. Evidence for such action is flimsy.
Administration: Parenteral.
Preparations: Multi-dose vial, 10 cc., 30 cc.
Dose: 1-2 cc.

DESERPIDINE—Harmonyl®
Tranquilizer. Rauwolfia material closely resembling reserpine in action. Used also in hypertension. Special merits yet to be established. Available in 0.1, 0.25 and 1.0 mg. tablets.

DESLANOSIDE—Cedilanid-D®
Cardiac stimulant. A digitalis material with much the same cardiac actions as lanatoside C, which see, but may be administered parenterally. Dosage also about the same. Replacing parenteral forms of lanatoside C.

DESOXYCORTICOSTERONE —Cortate®, Doca®, Percorten®
Adrenal cortical hormone. White crystalline powder, insoluble in water, usually the acetate or dimethylacetate.
Actions and Uses: One of the hormones of the cortex of the adrenal gland, chiefly concerned with the metabolism of salt and water. Useful in the management of chronic and acute insufficiency of the adrenal gland (Addison's disease of the adrenal gland).
Warnings: Overdosage may lead to edema, pulmonary congestion and signs of cardiac failure.
Administration: Intramuscular, implantation of pellets.
Preparations: Ampule, oily solution for parenteral administration. Pellet, for implantation. Vial, 10 cc. multi-dose.
Dose: 1-5 mg. daily, supplemented with sodium chloride for maintenance.

DESOXYEPHEDRINE®, see Methamphetamine

DESOXYN®, see Methamphetamine

DESSICATED THYROID EXTRACT, see Thyroid

DESYPHED®, see Methamphetamine

DEXEDRINE®, see Dextroamphetamine

DEXOVAL®, see Methamphetamine

DEXTRAN—Gentran®, Expandex®, Plavolex®
Parenteral fluid. A polysaccharide known as an expander.
Actions and Uses: Plasma substitute in treatment of shock.
Warnings: Inject slowly.
Administration: Intravenous.

Preparations: 6% in saline, in 500 cc. flasks.
Dose: As indicated by condition.

DEXTROAMPHETAMINE— d-AMFETASUL®, see Dextroam-
d-Amfetasul®, Dexedrine®
d-Amphetasul®, Dexedrine®
Stimulant (nervous system). Powder soluble in water, usually the sulfate.
Actions and Uses: Actions much the same as amphetamine but stimulates higher centers with less elevation of blood pressure. Used in treatment of obesity and psychologic depressions.
Warnings: Do not use in patients with hypertension or hyperexcitability.
Administration: Oral.
Preparations: Tablet, 5 mg.
Dose: 2.5 to 5 mg.

DEXTROMETHORPHAN— Romilar®
Cough suppressant. Dextroform of Racemorphan, the addictive analgesic. This form, however, is said to exert no euphoric effect and to have no addiction liability, but to retain, to a very high degree, the antitussive action of morphine. Clinical trial indicates that its antitussive action may be somewhat less than that of codeine; its final value is not yet established.

DEXTRO PROPOXYPHENE— Darvon®
Non-addictive analgesic. Relative usefulness remains to be established by long clinical trial. Available in 32 and 65 mg. capsules.

DEXTROSE—Glucose
Nutritional. White sweet powder, soluble in water.
Actions and Uses: A readily absorbed and utilized food and sugar which may be administered by virtually any route. It may also be used to sustain fluid volume when injected and to induce diuresis.
Warnings: Solutions are good media for bacterial growth; therefore reject all solutions which are not entirely clear, and maintain sterility.
Administration: Oral, intravenous, subcutaneous (hypodermoclysis), rectal.

Preparations: Solution in water, 5, 10, 20, 50%. Solution in saline, 5, 10, 20%.
Dose: Depends on indications.

DFP, see Isoflurophate

DIAFEN®, see Diphenylpyraline

DIAGNEX®, see Quinine Carbacrylic Resin

DIAL®, see Diallylbarbital

DIALLYLBARBITAL—Dial®
One of the intermediate acting barbiturates, which see.

DIAMINODIPHENYLSULFONE—
Avlosulfon®
Sulfone. New agent for treatment of leprosy.

DIAMOX®, see Acetazoleamide

DIAMTHAZOLE—Asterol®
Antifungal. New agent recommended for use in monilial and Trichophyton skin infections. Final position in the therapy of these resistant infections remains to be established. Available in 5% tincture and ointment.

DIAPARENE®, see Methylbenzethonium

DIAPHORETICS
Antipyretics, Pilocarpine.

DIASONE®, see Sulfoxone

DIATRINE®, see Methaphenilene

DIATRIZOATE—Hypaque®
Radio-opaque iodide. For diagnostic x-rays of urinary tract. Said to have low toxicity and to be excreted very rapidly by the kidneys after parenteral administration.

DIBASIC SODIUM PHOSPHATE,
see Sodium Phosphate

DIBENAMINE
Vasodilator. Formerly used in Raynaud's disease, little used at present.

DIBENZYLINE®, see Phenoxybenzamine

DIBUCAINE—Nupercaine®
Local and surface anesthetic. White crystals or powder with bitter taste, soluble in water.
Actions and Uses: Local anesthetic absorbed from the skin and mucous membranes and also effective after injection. More potent than cocaine or procaine.
Warnings: Considerably more toxic than either cocaine or procaine.
Administration: Intrathecal, tropical.
Preparations: Solution.
Dose: For spinal anesthesia, total dose should never exceed 12 mg. For local and surface anesthesia, 0.1%.

DICHLOROPHENARSINE—
Clorarsen®
Antiluetic. See Arsenic.

DICODID®, see Dihydrocodeinone

DICUMAROL®, see Bishydroxycoumarin

DICURIN®, see Merethoxylline

DICYCLOMINE—Bentyl®
Anticholinergic. White powder, usually the hydrochloride, soluble in water.
Actions and Uses: Antagonizes vagal tone in much the same way as atropine and has, therefore, the same therapeutic uses for peptic ulcer, intestinal hypermotility.
Warnings: Although stated to have less effect on eyes than atropine, the danger of glaucoma is, nevertheless, present.
Administration: Oral.
Preparations: Capsule, 10 mg. Syrup, 10 mg. per 4 cc.
Dose: 10 mg.

DIENESTROL, see Estrogens, Synthetic

DIETHYLCARBAMAZINE—Hetrazan®
Antifilarial.
Actions and Uses: For specific treatment of filariasis, loa loa, oncocerciasis and creeping eruption.
Warnings: A new drug, not well established as to either final value or dangers.
Administration: Oral.
Preparations: Tablet, 50 mg.
Dose: 2 mg. per Kg. body weight, 3 times daily.

DIETHYLSTILBESTROL—Stilbestrol, Stilphostrol®
Synthetic estrogen. White crystalline powder, insoluble in water.

Absorption: Well absorbed from G. I. tract.

Actions and Uses: Potent estrogenic drug which duplicates the actions of the natural estrogens and may be substituted for them for virtually all therapeutic purposes. May also be used in male in treatment of carcinoma of the prostate.

Warnings: May cause nausea and vomiting. In addition, indiscriminate use may produce, in common with other estrogens, excessive uterine bleeding.

Administration: Oral, intramuscular, subcutaneous.

Preparations: Capsule, tablet, 0.25, 0.5, 1.0 mg. Sterile solution.

Dose: Menopausal syndrome, 0.5 mg. daily. Carcinoma of prostate, much larger doses.

DIFFUSIN®, see Hyaluronidase

DIGILANID
Digitalis material. A mixture of glycosides from *Digitalis lanata*, relatively poorly absorbed from G. I. tract. More rapidly acting than digitalis leaf or digitoxin but otherwise much the same. See Digitalis.

DIGISEALS®, see Digitalis Leaf

DIGITALINE NATIVELLE®, see Digitoxin

DIGITALIS
In general, the principles are the same for all members of this group and the discussion of digitalis leaf below should, therefore, also apply to digitalis drugs which are not described here. The significant differences between the various members of the group are in speed of action and potency, hence dosage. Acetyldigitoxin, Acetylstrophanthidin, Cedilanid, Deslanoside, Digilanid, Digitalis, Digitoxin, Digoxin, Gitalin, Lanatoside C, Ouabain, Squill, Strophanthin.

DIGITALIS LEAF—Digiseals®, Digitora®
Cardiac stimulant.
The powdered leaf of *Digitalis purpurea*, a bitter greenish powder. Standardized by bio-essay, strength expressed in units

(cat, human, frog units, etc.) rather than weight. Contains a large proportion of impurities which, if given in full dosage at one time, may cause G. I. irritation, nausea and vomiting. Poorly absorbed, slowly eliminated, action develops slowly and is due to its digitoxin content which it resembles closely in its pharmacologic actions.

Actions and Uses: Typical of digitalis drugs.

Warnings: As for all digitalis materials; nausea and vomiting are usually the earlier signs of intoxication, visual disturbances and cardiac irregularity of more advanced intoxication. It is important, however, to distinguish these from similar symptoms caused by the patient's disease.

Preparations: Tablets, tincture, infusion, capsules, powder.

Dose: 0.1–0.2 Gm. (1 to 2 Units) daily as maintenance dose.

DIGITORA®, see Digitalis Leaf

DIGITOXIN—Crystodigin®, Digitaline Nativelle®, Purodigin®, Undigin®
Cardiac stimulant. A purified extract of digitalis leaf, with a slowly developing action and slow elimination (as long as two weeks after digitalization).

Warnings: As with all digitalis materials, watch for toxic symptoms. Parenteral solutions, often strongly alcoholic, may injure veins if injected without further dilution.

Administration: Oral, parenteral.

Absorption: Completely absorbed from G. I. tract.

Preparations: Tablet, usually coded: pink (0.1 mg.), white (0.2 mg.). Parenteral solution, 0.2 mg. per cc.

Dose: 0.1–0.2 mg. daily.

DIGLYCOCOLL HYDROIODIDE IODINE—Bursoline®
A soluble iodine compound used for the disinfection of drinking water.

DIGOXIN—Lanoxin®
Cardiac stimulant. A purified extract of *Digitalis lanata*. Relatively rapid devel-

opment of action and rapid elimination.
Administration: Oral, parenteral. Do not
inject parenteral solution intravenously
unless further diluted. Contains high
concentration of alcohol.
Dose: 0.5–1.0 mg. daily.

DIHYDROCODEINE—Rapacodin®
Addictive analgesic. Potency and usefulness relative to that of codeine remains to
be established by clinical trial. Available
in solution for parenteral use and 10 mg.
tablets.

DIHYDROCODEINONE—
Dicodid®, Paracodin®
Addictive analgesic. White powder, the
bitartrate, soluble in water.
Actions and Uses: The same as codeine
but somewhat more potent and more
addictive. See codeine.
Antidote: Nalorphine.

DIHYDROMORPHINONE—
Dilaudid®
Addictive analgesic. Derivative of mor-
phine.
Actions and Uses: Has all the properties
and disadvantages of morphine.
Warnings: See Morphine.
Administration: Oral, parenteral, rectal.
Preparations: Tablet, solution and sup-
pository.
Dose: 1–2.5 mg., depending in indica-
tions.
Antidote: Nalorphine.

DIHYDROSTREPTOMYCIN
Antibiotic. Usually the sulfate, white
crystals, soluble in water.
Actions and Uses: See Streptomycin.
Warnings: Has same disadvantages as
streptomycin with respect to rapid development of bacterial resistance. Less
toxic than streptomycin to vestibular ap-
paratus, which is the reason for its use
in preference to streptomycin but, on the
other hand, it is more likely to cause
deafness if its use is long continued.
Dose: Same order as streptomycin.

DIHYDROTACHYSTEROL—
Hytakerol®
A sterol which may be obtained from

ergosterol but without appreciable anti-
rachitic action, rather like that of parathyroid hormone. Used, therefore, in the
treatment of hypoparathyroidism.

DIHYDROTHEELIN, see Estradiol

**DIHYDROXYALUMINUM AMI-
NOACETATE**—Alglyn®, Alzi-
nox®, Aspogen®, Dimothyn®,
Doraxamin®, Robalate®
Antacid.
Actions and Uses: Buffers gastric acid,
in peptic ulcer and hyperacidity relieving
gastric pain without rebound acidity.
Warnings: Overuse may result in con-
stipation or obstipation.
Administration: Oral.
Preparations: Tablet, 0.5 Gm. Suspen-
sion, 0.5 Gm. per teaspoonful.
Dose: 1-2 tablets or teaspoonfuls.

DIHYDROXYANTHRAQUINONE
—Dorbane®
Cathartic. Purified anthraquinone compound; effective therefore, in small dosage (about 75 mg.), but providing no
particular advantage over cruder anthraquinone cathartics.

DIIODOHYDROXYQUINOLINE
—Diodoquin®, Moebiquin®,
Yodoxin®
Antiprotozoal. Colorless to tan powder,
usually odorless. Insoluble in water.
Actions and Uses: Drug of choice for
amebic dysentery, provided the amebae
have not extended beyond the intestine.
Also used in trichomonas intestinalis
infections.
Warnings: A safe drug, which may, how-
ever, cause chills, fever and skin erup-
tions.
Administration: Oral.
Preparations: Tablet, 0.2 Gm.
Dose: 1.5 Gm. for 2–3 weeks.

**DILANTIN®, see Diphenyl-
hydantoin**

**DILAUDID®, see Dihydromorph-
inone**

DILUTED HYDROCHLORIC ACID,
see Hydrochloric Acid

DIMENFORMON®, see Estradiol

DIMENHYDRINATE—Dramamine®
One of the large series of antihistamine drugs, which see. Said to be effective against nausea and vomiting and more especially in motion sickness. This action is apparently to be found in many others of the antihistamine drugs, in some better developed than in others.

DIMERCAPROL—BAL, British Anti-Lewisite
Heavy metal antidote. Colorless oily liquid with a skunk-like odor. Slightly soluble in water.
Actions and Uses: Protects vital enzyme systems of cells against effects of arsenic, mercury and gold poisoning; used in treatment of acute and chronic poisoning by these metals. Of less certain value in poisoning by other heavy metals.
Warnings: A disagreeable drug, which in the doses required in urgent cases of poisoning, may produce hypertension, nausea, vomiting, burning sensations of lips, severe headaches and sense of constriction in chest. Symptoms subside within about an hour. Cadmium poisoning may be aggravated by this drug.
Administration: Intramuscular, but may also be dissolved in water and used to wash the stomach and some may be permitted to remain in the stomach.
Preparations: Ampule, sterile solution in oil (10%), usually about 4.5 cc.
Dose: Maximum single dose, 5 mg. per Kg. body weight. Doses are always calculated on the basis of body weight, usually 3 mg. per Kg.

DIMETANE®, see Parabromdylamine

DIMETHICONE—Covicone®
Silicare®, Silicote®
Protective. A silicone derivative, which see, with skin-adherent and water-repellent properties, incorporated into ointments for skin protection.

DIMETHISOQUIN—Quotane®
One of the more potent surface anesthetics, which see.

DIMETHYLANE®, see Promoxolane

DIMETHYL-TUBOCURARINE—Mecostrin®, Metubine®
Skeletal muscle relaxant. See Tubocurarine.
Actions and Uses: Much the same as tubocurarine, which see.
Warnings: See Tubocurarine.
Antidote: Neostigmine.

DIMOTHYN®, see Dihydroxyaluminum Aminoacetate

DINACRIN®, see Isoniazid

DIOCTYL SODIUM SULFOSUCCINATE—Colace®, Diovac®,
Doxinate®, Molofac®
Stool softener.
Actions and Uses: A surface-active or wetting agent used in constipation to soften fecal material. Sometimes used in conjunction with laxative.
Warnings: New material, not yet clearly evaluated.
Administration: Oral, rectal.
Preparations: Capsules, 50 mg. liquid, 5 to 10 mg. per cc. syrup.
Dose: 1 to 2 capsules daily, 1 to 2 ounces in retention enema.

DIODOQUIN®, see Diiodohydroxyquinoline

DIODRAST®, see Iodopyracet

DIOGYN®, see Estradiol

DIOLOXOL®, see Mephenesin

DIONIN®, see Ethylmorphine

DIONOSIL®, see Propyliodine

DIOTHANE®, see Diperodon

DIOVAC®, see Dioctyl Sodium Sulfosuccinate

DIOXYLINE—Paveril®
Antispasmodic related to Papaverine, which see.

DI-PARALENE®, see Chlorcyclizine

DIPAXIN®, see Diphenadione

DIPERODON—Diothane®
One of the surface anesthetics. See Anesthetics, surface.

DIPHEMANIL—Prantal®
Anticholinergic.

Actions and Uses: Anticholinergic drug which relieves pain, favors healing, diminishes gastric motility and reduces gastric acidity in peptic ulcer. Also used in other intestinal spastic conditions as a substitute for atropine. Said to exert more effect on intestine and less on other structures than atropine.

Warnings: May cause mydriasis, dry mouth and elevated temperature. As with all members of this group, there is the danger of glaucoma in sensitive patients.

Administration: Oral.

Preparations: Tablet, 100 mg.

Dose: 100 mg. 3–4 times daily.

DIPHENADIONE—Dipaxin®

Anticoagulant. Related to Phenindione. One of the most potent and long-acting of the anticoagulants; effective in relatively small doses. Dosage of the order of 10 to 15 mg. daily with somewhat larger initial dosage. Prothrombin levels must be determined daily for safe use.

DIPHENHYDRAMINE—Benadryl®

One of the large series of antihistamine drugs, which see.

DIPHENYLHYDANTOIN —Dilantin®

Anticonvulsant. White powder, deteriorates on exposure to air. Freely soluble in water in the form of the sodium salt.

Absorption: Well absorbed from G. I. tract.

Actions and Uses: Controls grand mal and psychomotor seizures of epilepsy. May be of value in bronchial asthma, Parkinson's disease, chorea, and migraine, although not commonly used in these conditions.

Warnings: Nausea and vomiting, skin eruptions and soreness of the gums are relatively common. Central nervous system complications include disturbances in vision, ataxia, dizziness, tremors and psychoses.

Administration: Oral.

Preparations: Capsule, 30 mg., 100 mg.

Dose: Depends upon age and condition: Usually about 0.1 Gm. 3 times a day for an adult. Usually given after meals. This drug is often used for long periods of time, years in some cases. Given together with phenobarbital, effects may be enhanced.

DIPHENYLPYRALINE—Diafen®

Another of the long list of antihistamine drugs. More potent than most; the average dose is about 2 mg.

DIPROTRIZOATE SODIUM— Miokon®

Diagnostic. Radio-opaque iodide used for intravenous urography. 50% solution usually injected in doses of 20 to 30 cc. Reactions of warmth, nausea, urticaria, sweating and pain have been reported.

DIPYRONE—Methampyrone®, Narone®, Nartate®, Novaldin®

Non-addictive analgesic. Congener of aminopyrine; has all the dangers of bone-marrow depression of this series of drugs and should, therefore, be used with all appropriate precautions. See Aminopyrine. Available in 0.3 Gm. tablets and parenteral solution.

DISIPAL®, see Orphenadrine

DISULFIRAM—Antabuse®

Antialcoholic, metabolic.

Actions and Uses: Creates sensitivity to alcohol and produces extreme discomfort when patient under treatment ingests even small amounts of alcohol. Used as an adjunct in the treatment of alcoholism.

Warnings: A dangerous drug. Should be given only under close medical supervision. Should never be administered to a patient in a state of intoxication or without his full knowledge. Contraindicated in patients with or suspected of having coronary thrombosis or heart disease. Causes severe nausea and vomiting.

Administration: Oral.

Preparations: Tablet, 0.5 Gm.

Dose: Varies with patient sensitivity.

DITHRANOL®, see Anthralin

DITUBIN®, see Isoniazid

DIUCARDYN®, see Mercaptomerin

DIURETICS

Acetazoleamide, Aminometradine, Aminophylline, Amisometradine, Ammonium chloride, Chlormerodrin, Chlorothiazide, Meralluride, Mercaptomerin, Mercumantilin, Mercurophylline, Merethoxylline, Mersalyl, Theobromine calcium salicylate, Theobromine sodium acetate, Theobromine sodium salicylate, Theophylline sodium glycinate, Urea, Water.

DIURETIN®, see Theobromine and Sodium Salicylate

DIVINYL ETHER, see Vinyl Ether

d-LYSERGIC ACID, see Lysergic Acid Diethylamide

DOBELL'S SOLUTION, see Sodium Borate

DOCA®, see Desoxycorticosterone

DOLOPHINE®, see Methadon

DORAXAMIN®, see Dihydroxyaluminum Aminoacetate

DORBANE®, see Dihydroxyanthraquinone

DORIDEN®, see Glutethimide

DORMIN®, see Methapyrilene

DORMISON®, see Methylparafynol

DORSACAINE®, see Benoxinate

DORSAPHYLLIN®, see Theophylline Sodium Glycinate

DORYL®, see Carbachol

DOXINATE®, see Dioctyl Sodium Sulfosuccinate

DOXYFED®, see Methamphetamine

DOXYLAMINE—Decapryn®
One of the large series of antihistamine drugs, which see.

DRAMAMINE®, see Dimenhydrinate

DRISDOL®, see Synthetic Oleovitamin D

DROMORAN®, see Racemorphan

DUPONOL® BASE, see Duponol® Penetration Cream

DUPONOL® PENETRATION CREAM—Duponol® Base, So-

dium Lauryl Sulfate Cream
Vehicle.
Actions and Uses: A vehicle for drugs in which penetration of the pores of the skin and around hair follicles is desired. Used for oily skins in contrast to aerosol cream which is used for dry skins.
Warnings: Store in tightly stoppered containers.
Administration: Topical.

DURACILLIN®, see Penicillin

DURA-TAB
Proprietary name for a tablet which is so prepared as to confer an unusually prolonged action on any drug incorporated in it.

DYCLONE®, see Dyclonine

DYCLONINE—Dyclone®
Local anesthetic. Relatively new; uses, limitations and dangers not yet evaluated. Used in 0.5 to 1.0% concentration.

DYES
Colors (dyes) are harmless materials used to color fluid medications, often to disguise an unacceptable appearance, or because a particular color is recognized as a standard for a given preparation, or simply because of purely psychologic reasons.

E

ECOLID®, see Chlorisondamine

ECOTRIN®, see Acetylsalicylic Acid

ECTYLUREA—Nostyn®
Sedative and tranquilizer. New drug; value in either category should be questioned until established by long clinical trial. Available in 300 mg. tablets.

EDATHAMIL — EDTA, Calsol®, Sequestrene®, Versene®
Antidote. White soluble powder available as acid, sodium and calcium salts.
Absorption: Absorbed from the G. I. tract.
Actions and Uses: An entirely new kind

of drug, a so-called sequestering or chelating agent. This chemical literally draws certain metals from their combination with tissues, changes them into soluble and less toxic compounds, and accelerates their excretion from the body. EDTA is now used principally in lead poisoning but its final position in medicine is not yet determined and it is likely that this drug, or one like it, will be outstanding in the treatment of various types of metal poisoning. EDTA is especially important because lead poisoning is common and dimercaprol (BAL) is ineffectual in this condition.

Warnings: There is the possibility of hypocalcemia and tetany when the acid and the sodium salts of EDTA are used and, for that reason, the calcium salt is preferred. Inject slowly. In an unidentified poisoning or one in which the use of EDTA is not established there is the possibility that the combination between EDTA and the metal will not reduce toxicity.

Preparations: Ampules and tablets.
Dose: Intravenous, 1-2 Gm. in 250 cc. saline or dextrose solution. Oral, 30 mg. per Kg.
Antidote: Calcium.

**EDATHAMIL CALCIUM-DI-
SODIUM**—Calcium Disodium Versenate®
The preferred calcium disodium salt. See Edathamil.

EDIOL®, see Oral Fat Emulsion

EDROPHONIUM—Tensilon®
Antidote to curare. White crystalline powder, soluble in water and alcohol, usually the chloride.
Actions and Uses: Antagonizes curare and curare-like drugs; used, therefore, either to terminate curare effects when these are no longer necessary for therapeutic purposes or as an antidote in cases of overdosage or poisoning. Also for diagnosis in myasthenia gravis.
Warnings: In overdosage may intensify the curare effects. Should not be used in place of artificial respiration but as a

supplement to it. Because of parasympathomimetic actions may induce attacks of asthma. Should not be used as antidote to succinylcholine which it potentiates.
Administration: Intravenous.
Preparations: Vials, 10 cc., containing 10 mg. per cc.
Dose: 5 to 10 mg.

EDTA, see Edathamil

EFROXIN®, see Methamphetamine

**EFFERVESCENT PHOSPHATE
OF SODA, see Sodium Phosphate**

**EFFERVESCENT POWDERS,
COMPOUND**—Seidlitz Powders
Saline cathartic.
Actions and Uses: A sealed package containing two separate powders in papers, one which is blue and contains sodium bicarbonate and potassium sodium tartrate, and one paper which is white, which contains tartaric acid. The two are dissolved separately in about 2 ounces of water, and then mixed in a large glass. The mixture effervesces freely, and the mixture, which is a single dose, is then taken.
Warnings: The same as in the case of any cathartic.
Administration: Oral.

ELKOSIN®, see Sulfisomidine

ELORINE®, see Tricyclamol

EMETICS
Emetics are drugs which induce vomiting and used principally in treatment of poisoning. Two types are: (1) central emetics which act on the brain, and (2) local emetics which act on mucosa of stomach or intestinal tract.
Central emetics. Administered either orally or parenterally. Latter produces prompt results and is usually route of choice. Best known central emetic is apomorphine although morphine often produces same action in sensitive patients. Effects are produced in about a minute after injection of apomorphine.
Local emetics. Frequently used because of availability in the home. Because of irritant action they may be highly toxic

in large doses. It is well to remember this, especially when using a metalic emetic such as zinc or copper sulfate, which can cause serious poisoning. Should be used with great caution, never haphazardly, in considerable dilution. Apomorphine, Antimony potassium tartrate, Ipecac, Mustard (English).

EMETINE
Amebicide. White or yellowish crystalline powder, soluble in water, usually the hydrochloride. Slowly eliminated.

Actions and Uses: An effective antiamebic agent which is largely being displaced because it is more toxic and less effective than the more recent ones.

Warnings: Never inject intravenously. Continued use may cause central nervous system symptoms, cardiac disturbances, skin eruptions, hemoptysis, diarrhea, vomiting.

Administration: Intramuscular.

Preparations: Ampule, 1 cc. containing 20, 30, or 65 mg.

Dose: Given in courses, 65 mg. daily for about 10 days; 1–2 months should elapse between courses.

EMPERIN®
Analgesic. A proprietary mixture which consists of aspirin, acetophenetidin and caffeine, also commonly found in other widely advertised analgesic mixtures. There is also a form which contains codeine. At one time Emperin® contained aminopyrine, but at the present it does not.

Warnings: Whenever administering Emperin® it is well to read the label on the bottle to find out precisely what it contains.

ENTERO-VIOFORM®, see Iodochlorhydroxyquin

ENTROMONE®, see Gonadotropin, Chorionic

ENZEON®, see Chymotrypsin

ENZODASE®, see Hyaluronidase

EPHEDRINE—Racephedrine, I-sedrine®
Adrenergic and nasal decongestant. White

crystals, soluble in water, usually the sulfate.

Absorption: Well absorbed from G. I. tract.

Actions and Uses: Much the same as epinephrine (adrenalin), except it is considerably less potent. It elevates blood pressure, accelerates the heart and in large doses produces a sense of anxiety. Applied locally, it shrinks swollen nasal mucosa, and has, like epinephrine, an antiallergic action. Because of the last two, it is often used in hayfever and asthma. Effective in orthostatic hypotension. Unlike epinephrine, it is effective when taken by mouth.

Warnings: May elevate blood pressure excessively, cause headaches, nervousness, insomnia and spasm of the urinary bladder sphincter. Too frequent use may cause the development of resistance.

Administration: Oral, topical, parenteral.

Preparations: Capsule, 25, 50 mg. Syrup, for children, 4 mg. per 1 cc. Solution, sterile for injection, ampule or vial 50 mg. per 1 cc. Unsterile for topical administration, 0.25, 0.5, 1, 3%

Dose: 15-50 mg.

EPHENAMINE PENICILLIN G—
Compenamine®
Antibiotic.

Actions and Uses: New salt of penicillin with slow action of the same order as other repository penicillins; relatively low allergenicity. Not attended by any hazard of cross sensitization. Used in treatment of infections due to penicillin sensitive organisms in patients allergic to regular penicillin.

Administration: Intramuscular.

Preparations: Suspension in oil. Dry powder for aqueous suspension.

Dose: 300,000 Units.

EPINEPHRINE—Adrenalin®
Adrenergic. Usually obtained in solution, as the hydrochloride or tartrate.

Absorption: Not absorbed from G. I. tract. Destroyed and eliminated in body within about 5 minutes of injection.

Actions and Uses: As typical adrenergic, epinephrine duplicates most of the effects of stimulation of the sympathetic nervous system. Briefly, this includes acceleration of the heart, elevation of the blood pressure. Also produces a sense of anxiety. Applied to blood vessels, it causes constriction so that it tends to stop bleeding in wounds, and injected together with other drugs, it tends to delay their absorption into bloodstream. Has valuable antiallergic actions and may be used effectively in serious hypersensitivity reactions and intractable asthmatic attacks.

Warnings: May elevate blood pressure excessively, and in attacks of pulmonary edema due to cardiac disease, may be disastrous. Never inject the aqueous 1:100 solution.

Administration: Topical, inhalation of nebulae, parenteral.

Preparations: Solution, 1:1000, 1:100 for nebula only. Solution in oil, 1:500. Ophthalmic, solution, ointment.

Dose: Parenteral, 0.1–1.0 cc. of the 1:1000 solution.

EPSOM SALTS, see Magnesium Sulfate

EQUANIL®, see Meprobamate

ERGONOVINE—Ergotrate®
Oxytocic. White to yellow crystalline powder, moderately soluble in water, usually the maleate.

Absorption: Absorbed from G. I. tract.

Actions and Uses: Prompt and potent action on the uterus, causing it to contract. The effects which appear in a few minutes, may last for 3–4 hours. It is used as a routine measure after childbirth to prevent postpartum bleeding. It also may be used in the treatment of migraine headaches.

Warnings: Do not use in first and second stages of labor. May cause rupture of uterus and fetal asphyxia. Continued use may lead to gangrene.

Administration: Oral, intravenous, intramuscular.

Preparations: Tablet, 0.2 mg. Solution, 0.2 mg. per cc.

Dose: 0.2 mg.

ERGOT
Oxytocic. Purplish brown powder.

Absorption: Active ingredient absorbed from G. I. tract.

Actions and Uses: Causes potent contractions of uterus. This effect is utilized to limit postpartum bleeding and to prevent postpartum hemorrhage.

Warnings: Overdosage may cause gangrene. This is essentially the same condition caused by diseased rye called St. Anthony's Fire, ergot being the fungus which causes the disease of the rye. Ergot may not be used in the first and second stages of labor, during which it may cause rupture of uterus or asphyxia of fetus.

Administration: Oral.

Preparations: Extract, fluidextract, prepared ergot.

Dose: Varies with form used.

ERGOTAMINE—Gynergen®
Oxytocic. White crystals or powder, slightly soluble in water, usually the tartrate.

Absorption: Well absorbed from G. I. tract and sublingually.

Actions and Uses: Effective in producing uterine contractions much as ergot, but is largely used for a highly specific action in relief of migraine headaches. Latter action is presumed to be due to an action on the blood vessels within the skull.

Warnings: Continued use may cause gangrene in sensitive patients. Contraindicated in patients with nephritis, arteriosclerosis, hepatitis and scurvy. Toxicity may be increased in patients with hyperthyroidism. Frequently causes intense nausea in therapeutic doses.

Administration: Oral, sublingual, intramuscular.

Preparation: Sterile solution, 0.5 mg. per cc. Tablet, 1 mg.

Dose: 0.25–0.5 mg. by intramuscular route, 1.0 mg. by mouth.

ERGOTRATE®, see Ergonovine

ERIODICTYON—Yerba Santa
Flavor. Yellowish powder with aromatic odor.

Actions and Uses: Flavor used to make bitter taste.
Preparations: Fluidextract and aromatic syrup.
Dose: Fluidextract, 1 cc.; syrup, 8 cc.

ERYTHRITYL TETRANITRATE
—Erythrol tetranitrate
Vasodilator. Colorless and tasteless crystals. Explodes on percussion, but tablets made up with carbohydrate binder are nonexplosive.
Actions and Uses: Presumed to have a more prolonged action than nitroglycerin or amyl nitrite. Less potent than either and produces its effects much more slowly (about 30 minutes). See Nitrites.
Warnings: Continued use may cause methemoglobinemia. As with other nitrites, this drug may cause serious fall of blood pressure in overdosage. Protect from light and moisture.
Administration: Oral.
Preparations: Tablet, 15 mg., 30 mg.
Dose: 15–60 mg. every 5 hours.

ERYTHROCIN®, see Erythromycin

ERYTHROL TETRANITRATE, see Erythrityl Tetranitrate

ERYTHROMYCIN—Ilotycin®, Erythrocin®
Antibiotic. Available as crystals, ethyl carbonate, glucoheptonate, lactobionate, and stearate.
Absorption: Absorbed from G. I. tract.
Actions and Uses: New antibiotic obtained from *streptomyces erythreus,* effective against a wide variety of organisms. Does not destroy colon bacillus and therefore the normal flora of the bowel may be relatively unaffected. Early studies indicate no evidence of toxic effects. Especially valuable in staphyloccic infections because so many are now penicillin-resistant. Also effective against many rickettsial and large-virus infections.
Warnings: Continued clinical investigations are necessary before value of drug can be specifically determined.
Administration: Oral and parenteral.
Preparations: Tablet, 100 mg. Ampule, 250 mg. Solution, 100 mg. per teaspoonful.
Dose: 100–200 mg. 3 times daily.

ESERINE, see Physostigmine

ESOMID®, see Hexamethonium

ESTINYL®, see Ethinyl Estradiol

ESTRADIOL—Dihydrotheelin, Dimenformon®, Diogyn®, Ovocylin®, Progynon®
Estrogen. As such, the benzoate and dipropionate.
Administration: Oral, vaginal, percutaneous.
Preparations: Tablet, 0.1, 0.2, 0.5 mg. Ampule, 1.0 or 5.0 mg. per cc. in oil, or suppository, vaginal. Ointment.
Dose: 0.2 mg.

ESTRADIOL DIPROPIONATE
Estrogen.
Actions and Uses: See Estrogens.
Administration: Intramuscular.
Preparations: Ampule, sterile solution in sesame oil, containing 1.0 or 5.0 mg. per cc.
Dose: 1.0 mg. weekly.

ESTRADIOL VALERATE— Delestrogen®
Estrogen. Said to provide especially prolonged effects—2 to 3 weeks after a single injection. Value to be established by clinical trial. Available in 1 and 5 cc. vials.

ESTRADURIN®, see Polyestradiol Phosphate

ESTRIFOL®, see Estrogenic Substances, Conjugated

ESTRIOL—Theelol®, see Estrogens

ESTROGENIC SUBSTANCES, CONJUGATED—Amnestrogen®, Conestron®, Estrifol®, Hormesteral®, Konogen®, Premarin®
Estrogen. Obtained from pregnant mare urine, soluble in water.
Actions and Uses: See Estrogens.
Administration: Oral.
Preparations: Tablet, 0.3, 0.6, 1.25 and 2.5 mg.
Dose: As indicated by symptoms.

ESTROGENS

Estrogenic hormones represent a large number of natural and synthetic drugs, all of which have similar actions on the uterus, its lining, the vaginal epithelium, the mammary glands and the secondary sexual features of the female. In addition they exert a specific restraining action on carcinoma of the prostate of the male.

The natural estrogens may be recovered from the ovary, the urine of pregnant humans and pregnant animals, and the placenta. These include impure mixtures as well as chemical derivatives of these natural estrogens such as estradiol benzoate and ethinyl estradiol.

The synthetic materials such as stilbestrol, produce essentially the same effects as natural estrogens, but it is said that side effects and minor toxic actions may be more common with the synthetic materials.

The gravest danger in the continued and improper scheduling of the dosage with estrogens is uterine hypertrophy and bleeding, an action which often leads to an erroneous suspicion of uterine carcinoma.

The commonest indication for estrogen therapy is menapause, but they are used also for disorders of vaginal mucosa dysmenorrhea, prostatitis and mammary and prostatic carcinoma.

The drugs, depending on which one is used, may be taken orally or parenterally and may be given in conjunction with androgenic hormones.

The dosage is variable and depends on the material, the symptoms and response to therapy. Overdosage or too long continued use in the female may cause severe menstrual bleeding.

Natural estrogens: Estradiol; Estriol; Estrogenic substances, conjugated; Estrone, Polyestradiol.

Synthetic estrogens: Benzestrol, Chlorotriansene, Dienestrol, Diethylstilbestrol, Hexestrol, Mestilbol, Methallenestril, Promethestrol.

ESTRONE—Estrugenone®, Estrusol®, Sulestrex®, Theelin®, Thelestrin®
Estrogen.
Actions and Uses: See Estrogens.
Administration: Intramuscular, oral.
Preparations: Ampule, sterile solution in sesame oil containing 1.0 or 5.0 mg. per cc. Tablet, 1.25 mg.
Dose: 0.2–1.0 mg. weekly.

ESTRUGENONE®, see Estrone

ESTRUSOL®, see Estrone

ETAMON®, see Tetraethylammonium

ETHCHLORVYNOL—Placidyl®
Another of the very recent hypnotic drugs. Not a barbiturate, but its advantages over the latter remain to be proven.
Preparations: Capsule, 0.5 Gm.
Dose: Of the order of 0.5 Gm.

ETHER—Ethyl Ether
Anesthetic and solvent. A colorless fluid, with a characteristic odor, volatile and inflammable.
Actions and Uses: By inhalation, absorbed through the lungs and depresses the central nervous system producing sleep, loss of pain appreciation, and loss of reflexes. Action depends on its concentration in the blood. One of the safest anesthetics because serious depression of the vital centers occurs late in anesthesia.
Warnings: Inflammable and mixtures with air are explosive although much less so than cyclopropane. Overdosage may cause depression of respiration. Should be stored in tight containers, at a reduced temperature and away from light.
Administration: Inhalation, drops, mask, machine.
Preparations: Liquid.
Dose: This is a variable which is under the control of the anesthetist.

ETHINAMATE—Valmid®
Hypnotic. One of the new hypnotic agents for which great stress is being laid on the fact that it is not a barbiturate. Whether it will prove to have any

advantages either therapeutically or from the point of view of toxic reactions remains to be seen. There is no reason to believe that, in the relief of anxiety, it presents less hazard of habituation than the barbiturates.
Preparations: Tablet, 0.5 Gm.
Dose: Of the order of 0.5-1.0 Gm. orally.

ETHINYL ESTRADIOL—Estinyl®, Eticylol®, Lynoral®, Oradiol®, Orestralyn®
Estrogen, which see. Absorbed from G.I. tract, administered orally.

ETHIODOL®, see Iodinated Poppyseed Oil

ETHISTERONE—Lutocylol®, Pranone®, Anhydroxyhydroprogesterone
Corpus luteum hormone. Synthetic material. White or yellow crystals, insoluble in water.
Absorption: Absorbed from G. I. tract.
Actions and Uses: Said to be of value in dysmenorrhea, premenstrual tension and in habitual abortion.
Warnings: Overdose may cause headache, fainting and prolonged weakness.
Administration: Oral.
Preparations: Tablet, 10 mg., 25 mg.
Dose: 10-25 mg. daily.

ETHOPROPAZINE—Parsidol®
Muscle relaxant. The hydrochloride.
Actions and Uses: One of the new skeletal muscle relaxants which has been recommended for the treatment of muscle rigidity in Parkinson's Disease. Also said to relieve psychic tensions. Final position yet to be established.
Preparations: Tablet, 10 mg.
Dose: Of the order of 100-200 mg. daily.

ETHOTOIN—Peganone®
Anticonvulsant. For grand mal seizures. Closely related to Diphenylhydantoin, which see. Available in 0.25 and 0.5 Gm. tablets.

ETHYL ALCOHOL, see Alcohol

ETHYL AMINOBENZOATE
—Anesthesin®, Benzocaine®
Surface anesthetic. White crystals or powder relatively insoluble in water.
Absorption: Absorbed from skin, mucous membranes and wounds.
Actions and Uses: Produces local anesthesia. Used in relief of superficial pain from skin eruptions, burns, etc.
Warnings: May cause dermatitis. Excessive amounts applied topically, especially on broken skin or mucous surfaces, may result in absorption with systemic toxic effects.
Administration: Topical.
Preparations: Lozenge, 0.1 Gm. Ointment, 10%. Suppository, 0.2 Gm.
Dose: Concentration, 1-10%.

ETHYL BISCOUMACETATE—
Tromexan®
Anticoagulant.
A coumarin derivative, more potent and more rapid in its curve of action than bishydroxycoumarin (Dicumarol®) but with no other established advantages either in therapeutic effects or decreased toxicity or increased ease of application. Dosage five to six times as large as bishydroxycoumarin, which see.

ETHYL CHLORIDE
Local anesthetic and refrigerant. Colorless and volatile liquid. Inflammable.
Actions and Uses: Has long been used as a general anesthetic, but has largely been discarded for this purpose. When sprayed on the skin, its rapid evaporation results in intense refrigeration. This action can be used to produce local anesthesia, and in addition, by a reflex, may also relieve deeper muscle pains.
Warnings: Excessive refrigeration may produce serious local damage.
Administration: Topical spray.
Preparations: A special stoppered bottle, so that it delivers a spray which can be controlled. The power for the spray is produced by the extreme volatility of the liquid.
Dose: As indicated by condition.

ETHYLENE
Anesthetic. Colorless gas with sweet odor. Inflammable and explosive.
Actions and Uses: Same as ether. More pleasant for the patient to take. Its use

has been largely discontinued because of the grave danger of explosion.
Warnings: Mixtures with air are explosive.
Administration: Inhalation.
Preparations: Gas through closed inhalation machine.
Dose: As with any volatile anesthetic, determined by anesthetist.

ETHYLENEDIAMINE
Solvent. A slightly yellow liquid. Miscible with water.
Actions and Uses: As a solvent, especially for xanthine drugs, e.g. theophylline. Toxicity is very low.

ETHYL ETHER, see Ether

ETHYLMORPHINE—Dionin®
Addictive analgesic. White or yellow powder, soluble in water, usually the hydrochloride.
Actions and Uses: Similar to morphine and codeine and intermediate in potency. Largely displaced, since it has no advantages over either. Applied to the eye, it produces local vasodilation which is, perhaps, its most important use at present.
Warnings: See Morphine.
Administration: Oral, topical (in eye).
Preparations: Ophthalmic solution, ointment, 5–10%. Tablet, 15 mg., 30 mg.
Dose: Oral, 15-30 mg. for cough. Topical, 5-10% concentration.
Antidote: Nalorphine.

ETHYLNOREPINEPHRINE—
Bronkephrine®
Adrenergic. Said to resemble Isoproterenol in its actions, which see, and recommended largely for the relief of asthmatic symptoms. Applied either intravenously or intramuscularly in doses of about 2 mg.

ETHYLSTIBAMINE—
Neostibosan®
An antimony compound with much the same uses, dangers and dosage of Stibamine glucoside, which see.

ETICYLOL®, see Ethinyl Estradiol

EUCATROPINE—Euphthalamine®

Mydriatic, anticholinergic. White powder soluble in water, the hydrochloride.
Actions and Uses: Dilates pupils promptly without increasing intraocular tension, causing pain, irritation or anesthesia of the conjunctiva.
Warnings: May cause acute glaucoma in sensitive patients.
Administration: Topical.
Preparations: Solution.
Dose: 2-3 drops of a 5% solution.

EUGENOL
Surface anesthetic. Yellow liquid with characteristic odor.
Actions and Uses: Same as clove oil, in dentistry, by local application in cavities of teeth to reduce pain.
Warnings: Overdosage may produce intestinal irritation.
Administration: Topical.
Preparations: Oil. ·
Dose: 0.1 cc.

EUPHTHALAMINE®, see Eucatropine

EURAX®, see Crotamiton

EVIPAL®, see Hexobarbital

EXCHANGE RESINS
A group of relatively inert materials, which have no direct action on the body or its functions. They do, however, combine with acid or alkaline ions (depending on the type used) and hold them tenaciously. Thus, if such substances are given together with food, they will remove from it, acid or alkali, as the case may be. If the cationic resins, namely those which combine with alkaline materials are given together with with food, they will remove principally sodium. Thus, it becomes possible, with their use, to give a patient a diet which is flavored with sodium chloride, and yet to treat it in such a way, that the sodium chloride does not get into the system. This device, therefore, is a way around the salt-poor diet, which is such a hardship for so many cardiac patients. The disadvantages of these substances are: (1) disagreeable texture, making it difficult to take; (2) limited ability to

remove salt, so that full freedom to take salt may not be granted; (3) removes other important alkaline ions, principally potassium and calcium, but there are some resins which provide these ions in excess to overcome this objection; (4) cause gastric distress in many patients; (5) may cause serious constipation. Other exchange resins combine with acids and are used to counteract the gastric acid in patients who are being treated for peptic ulcers. They are not as desirable as the antacids which are so much more commonly used, principally because of their irritant action on the intestinal tract and their tendency to produce constipation.

Sodium removing: Carbacrylamine, Carboxylic, and Styronate resins.

Acid removing: Polyamine-methylene, and Quinine Carbacrylic Resins.

EXORBIN®, see Polyamine-methylene Resins

EXPANDEX®, see Dextran

EXPECTORANTS
Ammonium chloride, Ammonium carbonate, Hydriodic acid, Ipecac, Potassium iodide. Terpin hydrate.

EXTENTAB
Proprietary name for a tablet which is so prepared as to confer an unusually prolonged action on any drug incorporated in it.

F

FARGAN®, see Promethazine

F-CORTEF®, see Fludrocortisone

FEOSOL®, see Ferrous Sulfate

FERGON®, see Ferrous Gluconate

FERRIC AMMONIUM CITRATE
Hematinic. Reddish scales, granules or powder, soluble in water.
Absorption: Absorbed from G. I. tract.
Actions and Uses: For treatment of iron deficiency anemia.
Warnings: Tends to cause G. I. distress and has largely been displaced by ferrous

salts. In common with all iron salts, turns stools dark green or black. May cause diarrhea.
Administration: Oral, parenteral.
Preparations: Capsule, 0.5 Gm. Sterile solution.
Dose: Oral, 1 Gm. Parenteral, 0.1 Gm.

FERRIC CACODYLATE
Hematinic.
Actions and Uses: An iron compound which contains arsenic and is rarely used today. See Iron and Arsenic.

FERRIC CHLORIDE
Astringent. Orange crystals.
Actions and Uses: Used mainly as an astringent, rarely as an hematinic.
Warnings: Highly irritant. May injure teeth.
Administration: Topical.
Preparations: Tincture, 13% ferric chloride.
Dose: Local application of the tincture as indicated.

FERRIC GLYCEROPHOSPHATE
Hematinic.
Actions and Uses: Has no advantages over ordinary iron salts and not commonly used today. See Iron.

FERRIC HYPOPHOSPHITE
Hematinic.
Actions and Uses: No advantages over ordinary iron salts and not commonly used today. See Iron.

FERRIC PHOSPHATE
Hematinic.
Actions and Uses: Has the same disadvantages of the other ferric salts as an hematinic. Not commonly used today. See Iron.

FERRONORD®, see Iron Glycamine

FERROUS CARBONATE
Hematinic. Brownish powder or mass.
Absorption: From G. I. tract.
Actions and Uses: In common with other iron salts. Useful in treatment of iron deficiency anemia. Its use is decreasing in favor of the sulfate. See Iron.
Warnings: May irritate G. I. tract. Better tolerated if given after meals.

Administration: Oral.
Preparations: Mass, containing honey and sugar. Pill, Blaud's pills. Saccharated.
Dose: 0.6 Gm.

FERROUS GLUCONATE
Hematinic.
Actions and Uses: May be less irritating to G. I. tract and, therefore, generally used as a substitute for ferrous sulfate in cases in which the ferrous sulfate cannot be tolerated. See Iron.
Administration: Oral.
Preparations: Tablet, 0.3 Gm. which represents 35 mg. of iron.
Dose: 0.3 Gm.

FERROUS IODINE
Hematinic. The combination with iodine provides no advantage over the iron or iodine alone in situations where either is indicated, or a combination in cases in which both are indicated. Rarely used.

FERROUS SULFATE—
Feosol®
Hematinic. Green crystals or granules, soluble in water.
Absorption: From G. I. tract.
Actions and Uses: Effective hematinic in iron deficiency anemia. Presumably more effective and less irritant than equivalent amounts of ferric salts. See Iron.
Warnings: May cause G. I. distress, diarrhea. Best taken immediately after eating. Stools turn dark green or black. Store in dry place.
Administration: Oral.
Preparations: Tablet, 0.2 Gm. or 0.3 Gm., usually coated. Syrup. Elixir.
Dose: Modern dosage is rather large, eg., 0.2-0.6 Gm. 3-4 times daily. See Iron.

FIBRIN FOAM
Hemostatic. Sponge-like material.
Actions and Uses: Acts as mechanical agent as well as accelerating blood clotting to stop bleeding.
Administration: Directly, with pressure, if necessary with thrombin.
Preparations: Package containing 250 mg. fibrin foam, together with vial of thrombin.

Dose: Use amount necessary to stop bleeding.

FIBRINOGEN (HUMAN)
Hemostatic. Prepared from human plasma and injected to restore blood fibrinogen levels to normal after extensive surgery, in diseases, or hemorrhagic complications with afibrinogenemia. Not to be used instead of whole-blood when formed elements are needed, though it provides more fibrinogen than possible with whole-blood transfusions. The risk of transfusion hepatitis is somewhat greater than with whole-blood transfusion.

FLAXEDIL®, see Gallamine

FLAXSEED, see Linseed

FLEXIBLE COLLODION, see Collodion, Flexible

FLEXIN®, see Zoxazolamine

FLORINEF®, see Fludrocortisone

FLOROPRYL®, see Isoflurophate

FLUDROCORTISONE—Alflorone®,
F-Cortef®, Florinef®
Anti-inflammatory hormone. A hydrocortisone derivative containing fluorine. It is more potent than hydrocortisone by topical application and, although it is stated to be less likely to produce systemic effects, these have already been reported after its local application. The indications for its use and the precautions to be taken are the same as in the case of hydrocortisone, which see. Available in 0.1 and 0.2% ointments and lotions.

FLUORESCEIN SODIUM
Diagnostic dye.
Actions and Uses: Used to determine circulation time, or state of circulation in damaged skin or corneal surface.
Warnings: Use local anesthetic before applying directly to cornea.
Administration: Intravenous, topical.
Preparations: Solution, for injection 20%; for topical use, 1-2%.
Dose: Intravenous, 2.5 cc. Eye drops, 2-3 drops.

FLUOXYMESTRONE—Halotestin®
Androgen. Claimed to have outstanding potency by the oral route and be able to replace parenteral testosterone therapy. Value yet to be established. Available in 2 and 5 mg. tablets.

FOLIC ACID—Folvite®
Hematinic. Yellow-orange powder, insoluble in water. Sodium salt available.
Absorption: From the G. I. tract.
Actions and Uses: In pernicious anemia, used to supplement liver therapy. Increases number of red cells and hemoglobin content and acts in much the same way as liver itself, but does not prevent the neurologic complications of pernicious anemia. Also of value in other conditions in which liver extract is used. Controls the diarrhea of sprue.
Warnings: Should not be substituted for liver extracts in pernicious anemia. Of no value in aplastic anemia or iron deficiency anemia.
Administration: Oral, intramuscular.
Preparations: Capsule, tablet, 5–10 mg. (tablets may be scored). Ampule, containing powder to be dissolved before using, 15 mg.
Dose: 2.5–20 mg.

FOLLUTEIN®, see Gonadotropin, Chorionic

FOLVITE®, see Folic Acid

FORMALDEHYDE—Formalin
Disinfectant. A highly irritant clear solution with a characteristic irritant odor.
Actions and Uses: Solution and vapors may be used for disinfection of instruments, drapes, etc., but commonly for rooms. Also used directly on skin to harden it and to reduce sweating.
Warnings: Highly toxic and irritant. Not to be taken internally.

FORMALIN, see Formaldehyde

FORTHANE®, see Methylhexaneamine

FOWLER'S SOLUTION, see Potassium Arsenite

FOXGLOVE, see Digitalis

FRENQUEL®, see Azacyclonal

FRUCTOSE—Levulose, Levugen®
Nutritional. A sugar occuring naturally in fruits; soluble, sweet, recently introduced.
Actions and Uses: Said to be more readily available for utilization after infusion than dextrose. Has had little use because of newness.
Administration: Intravenous.
Preparations: Solution, 10% in 1000 cc. flasks.
Dose: As indicated.

FUADIN®, see Stibophen

FUGILLIN®, see Fumagillin

FUMAGILLIN—Fugillin®, Fumidil®
Amebicide. Antibiotic derived from Aspergillus fumigatus.
Absorption: From G.I. tract.
Actions and Uses: Potent amebicide, used both in man and animals infected with E. histolytica and in other forms of human amebiasis.
Warnings: Ineffective against most bacteria, fungi and viruses, useless in common dysenteries, virtually specific for amebiasis. Nausea, vomiting, anorexia, diarrhea have been reported. Examine blood regularly and observe for effects on liver and kidneys.
Administration: Oral.
Preparations: Capsule, 10 mg.
Dose: 10 to 60 mg. daily.

FUMIDIL®, see Fumagillin

FUMING NITRIC ACID, see Nitric Acid, Fuming

FURACIN®, see Nitrofurazone

FURADANTIN®, see Nitrofurantoin

FURAZOLIDONE—Furoxone®
Antiseptic, trichomonacide. Nitrofuran derivative. Used by topical application in relief of trichomonas vaginitis. Supplied in 0.25% suppositories and 0.1% powder.

FURMETHIDE®, see Furtrethonium

FUROXONE®, see Furazolidone

FURTRETHONIUM—Furmethide®
Cholinergic. White powder, the iodide, soluble in water.
Actions and Uses: Much the same actions and effects as methacholine but said to exert a much more intense effect on the urinary bladder and less on other systems, and hence, used in urinary retention. See Methacholine.
Warnings: May set off attacks of asthma in patients with previous history of asthma. Keep atropine on hand when using.
Administration: Oral, subcutaneous.
Preparations: Tablet, 10 mg. Ampule, 5 mg. in 1 cc.
Dose: 1–5 mg.
Antidote: Atropine.

G

GALACTOSE
Diagnostic. White powder.
Absorption: From G. I. tract.
Actions and Uses: Used for liver function test. When liver is normal no galactose appears in the urine after an oral dose. When liver is badly damaged some of the sugar appears unchanged in the urine.
Warnings: Solution must be freshly prepared. Do not dissolve sugar with heat.
Administration: Oral.
Preparations: Vial, containing 40 Gm.
Dose: 40 Gm.

GALLAMINE—Flaxedil®
Skeletal muscle relaxant.
Actions and Uses: Synthetic substitute for tubocurare, which see. Used in anesthesia and shock therapy in much the same way.
Warnings: Overdosage may lead to respiratory paralysis; tends to accelerate heart rate.
Administration: Intravenous.
Preparations: 20 cc. vials, solution 20 mg. per cc.
Dose: 20 mg. per 45 lbs. body weight.

GALLOTANNIC ACID, see Tannic Acid

GAMBOGE
Cathartic. A drastic cathartic, now used only in veterinary medicine.

GAMMA BENZENE HEXACHLORIDE, see Benzene Hexachloride, Gamma

GAMOPHEN,®, see Hexachlorophene

GANTRISIN®, see Sulfisoxazole

GANTRISIN® ACETYL, see Acetyl Sulfisoxazole

GASTRIC MUCIN—Mucin
Protectant. White to yellow powder or drugs, which see.
granules, slightly bitter taste; forms opalescent solution with water.
Actions and Uses: Protective in treatment of peptic ulcer, usually in mixtures with antacids or other medicaments.
Administration: Oral.
Preparations: Powder and granules.
Dose: 2.5 Gm., usually at 2 hour intervals.

GELATIN
Foodstuff. White to yellowish sheets or flakes.
Actions and Uses: Food and vehicle or base. Also available in special form for intravenous use as a plasma expander.
Warnings: Sometimes contains tetanus spores. Use only special material for intravenous injection.

GELATIN FILM, ABSORBABLE—Gelfilm®
A gelatin film used in surgical repair of membranes.

GELATIN SPONGE, ABSORBABLE—Gelfoam®
Hemostatic.
Actions and Uses: A surgical sponge used to control bleeding which may be left in situ without causing a reaction.

GELFILM®, see Gelatin Film, Absorbable

GELFOAM®, see Gelatin Sponge, Absorbable

GEMONIL®, see Metharbital

GENTIAN
Flavor. Yellow to brown powder with bitter taste.
Actions and Uses: Has local action on stomach and bitter taste which may combine to stimulate appetite.
Warnings: Excessive dose may cause nausea and vomiting.
Administration. Oral.
Preparations: Elixir, glycerinated elixir, extract, fluidextract, and most frequently, the compound tincture of gentian 10% (which also contains aromatic flavors, glycerin and alcohol).
Dose: 4 cc. of the compound tincture.

GENTIAN VIOLET, see Methylrosaniline

GENTRAN®, see Dextran

GEXANE®, see Benzene Hexachloride, Gamma

GINEBATIN®, see Bacitracin

GINGER
Flavor.
Actions and Uses: Because of its aromatic odor and its irritating action on the stomach, it is used as a stimulant to G. I. tract.
Preparations: Fluidextract, oleoresin, syrup.
Dose: 0.6 Gm.

GITALIGIN®, see Gitalin

GITALIN—Gitaligin®
A digitalis material, which see.

GLAUBER'S SALT, see Sodium Sulfate

GLOBIN ZINC INSULIN
One of the slowly acting forms of insulin, which see.

GLUCOPHYLLINE®, see Theophylline-Methylglucamine

GLUCOSE, see Dextrose

GLUCOSULFONE—Promin®
Sulfone. Used principally in the treatment of leprosy, but also as an adjunct in the treatment of tuberculosis. Reac-

tions occur in about 10% of patients. Intravenous dose is about 2 to 5 Gm. daily for 6 days and repeated after a rest period only.

GLUCURONE®, see Glucuronolactone

GLUCURONOLACTONE—Glucurone®
Anti-arthritic. Value and dangers yet to be established by long clinical trial. Available in 0.5 Gm. tablets.

GLUTAMIC ACID
Anticonvulsant. White crystalline powder, soluble in water, also sodium salt.
Absorption: From G. I. tract.
Actions and Uses: Formerly used in combination with other medication in treatment of epileptic seizures. Rarely used now.
Warnings: Ineffective against grand mal seizures.
Administration: Oral.
Preparations: Powder.
Dose: 1 Gm.

GLUTAMIC ACID HYDROCHLORIDE—Acidoride®, Acidulin®, Glutan®, Hydrionic®
Digestive.
Actions and Uses: Releases hydrochloric acid on contact with water, providing this acid in the stomach for cases of gastric hypoacidity. Chief advantage is convenience of administration over that of diluted hydrochloric acid.
Administration: Oral.
Preparations: Capsule; equivalent of 10 minims of diluted hydrochloric acid.
Dose: 1-3 capsules 3 times daily.

GLUTAN®, see Glutamic Acid Hydrochloride

GLUTAVENE®, see Sodium Glutamate

GLUTETHIMIDE—Doriden®
Hypnotic. A new drug introduced with major emphasis on the fact that it is not a barbiturate. Effectiveness as a hypnotic as compared with barbiturates remains to be determined but there is no reason

to believe that dangers of habituation are less. Available in 250 and 500 mg. tablets.

GLYCERIN
Vehicle. Clear colorless fluid with a sugary taste.
Actions and Uses: As a vehicle, and externally for its emollient action on the skin. Has a mildly irritant action on rectal mucosa which is the basis for its use in the glycerine suppository.

GLYCERITE OF HYDROGEN PEROXIDE®, see Carbamide Peroxide

GLYCEROPHOSPHATES
Actions and Uses: A group of salts, sodium, iron, calcium, manganese, which for a long time have been recommended and widely used as a nerve tonic. There is no evidence that any of the claims made for the glycerophosphates are founded on fact. Usually the mixtures have a winey flavor and a fairly high alcoholic content in order to make them more attractive.

GLYCERYL TRINITRATE—Nitroglycerin, Nitroglyn®
Vasodilator. A highly explosive liquid, but when dispensed in tablets with a lactose base, there is no such danger.
Absorption: Rapidly absorbed from mucous membrane of tongue.
Actions and Uses: Dilates small arterioles by relaxing, lowering the blood pressure.
Warnings: May cause severe headaches if dose is too large. Tablets are unstable, and old ones should not be used. Hypo tablets, rather than compressed tablets, should be used.
Administration: Sublingual, oral.
Preparations: Tablet.
Dose: 0.3–0.6 mg.

GLYCINE, see Aminoacetic Acid

GLYCOBIARSOL—Milibis®
Antiprotozoal. Yellowish crystals slightly soluble in water. Arsenical.
Actions and Uses: An amebicide used only in treatment of amebic infestations of intestine. See Arsenic.

Warnings: An arsenical possessing same dangers as other arsenicals as well as of bismuth.
Administration: Oral.
Preparations: Tablet 0.25 Gm.
Dose: 0.5 Gm.
Antidote: Dimercaprol.

GLYCOCHOLIC ACID, see Ox Bile Extract

GLYCOCOLL, see Aminoacetic Acid

GLYCYRRHIZA—Licorice Root
Flavor.
Preparations: Extract, fluidextract, syrup.
Actions and Uses: A flavoring agent.

GLYCYRRHIZA COMPOUND, see Senna

GLYNAZAN®, see Theophylline Sodium Glycinate

GLYTHEONATE®, see Theophylline Sodium Glycinate

GOLD
Until cortisone was introduced gold salts were the most effective specific drugs in treatment of rheumatoid arthritis. These drugs helped many patients, failed with others. Because of their high index of toxicity gold salts required long experience before they could be used with relative safety. Only extreme distress of arthritis warranted the use of these drugs. Toxic effects have been: agranulocytosis, alopecia (baldness), anemia, bronchitis, conjunctivitis, diarrhea, dermatitis, erythema, gingivitis, nephritis, hepatitis. Dimercaprol is the drug of choice in treating reactions to gold salts. Aurothioglucose, Aurothioglycanide, Gold sodium thiomalate, Gold sodium thiosulfate.

GOLD SODIUM THIOMALATE—Myochrysine®
Antiarthritic.
Actions ad Uses: Used in treatment of rheumatoid arthritis and lupus erythematosus.
Warnings: See Gold.
Administration: Intramuscular.
Preparations: Ampule, 10, 25, 50, 100 mg. per cc.

Dose: Maximum of 25 mg. per week.
Antidote: Dimercaprol.

GOLD SODIUM THIOSULFATE
Antiarthritic.
Actions and Uses: Chemotherapeutic agent used in treatment of rheumatoid arthritis, lupus erythematosus and psoriasis.
Warnings: See Gold.
Administration: Intravenous, intramuscular.
Preparations: Ampule, containing crystals to be made up into solutions before using. 10, 25, 50, 100, 250 mg.
Dose: Usually in graded doses up to 25 mg. weekly, until a total of 1-1.5 Gm. has been given.
Antidote: Dimercaprol.

GONADOTROPIN, CHORIONIC—
Entromone®, Follutein®
Gonadotropic hormone. Powder, unstable in solution.
Actions and Uses: Cryptorchism, hypogonadism, uterine bleeding. Its value in all but cryptochism remains to be established.
Warnings: Excessive dosage may induce pseudo-puberty, and precocious sexuality.
Administration: Parenteral.
Preparations: Vial, 10 cc., containing 5,000 or 10,000 Units.
Dose: 500 to 1000 Units twice weekly.

G-PENICILLIN, see Penicillin

GRAMACIDIN—Gramoderm®
Antibiotic. Used only topically for superficial infections. Available as an ointment.

GRAMODERM®, see Gramacidin

GREEN, BRILLIANT, see Brilliant Green

GREEN, SOAP, see Soap, Medicinal, Soft

G-STROPHANTHIN, see Ouabain

GUAIACOL
Antiseptic. Colorless to yellow solid or liquid, with aromatic odor.
Actions and Uses: Antiseptic and bronchial stimulant.
Warnings: Large doses may be highly irritant.

Administration: Topical, oral.
Preparations: Mixtures with other medicaments.
Dose: 0.5 c.c.

GUANATOL®, see Chloroguanide

GUM ARABIC, see Acacia

GUM MYRRH, see Myrrh

GUM TRAGACANTH, see Tragacanth

GYNERGEN®, see Ergotamine

H

HALAZONE
Antiseptic. White powder, chlorine odor, slightly soluble in water.
Actions and Uses: Disinfection of drinking water.
Preparations: Tablet, 4 mg.
Dose: 4 to 8 mg. per liter of water.

HALIBUT LIVER OIL
Vitamin. Fishy oil from livers of halibut.
Actions and Uses: Source of vitamin A and D, usually for infant feeding and prophylaxis.
Warnings: Store in a cool place and protect from direct light.
Administration: Oral.
Preparations: Capsule, 0.2 cc. (about 5000 Units vitamin A and 85 Units vitamin D).
Dose: 1-2 capsules daily.

HALOTESTIN®, see Fluoxymestrone

HARD SOAP, see Soap, Hard

HARMONYL®, see Deserpidine

HARTMANN'S SOLUTION, see Lactated Ringer's Solution

HASHISH, see Cannabis

HEDULIN®, see Phenindione

HELIUM
Gas. Used with oxygen as a less dense substitute for air, with decreasing effort required for respiration in high altitudes and various types of dyspnea. Used with Cyclopropane to decrease its flammability.

HELLEBORE, see Veratrum Viride

HEMATINICS
Arsenic Trioxide, Folic acid, Iron compounds, Iron-Dextran, Liver, Stomach preparations, Vitamin B_{12}

HEMO-PAK®, see Cellulose, Oxidized

HENBANE, see Hyoscyamus

HEPARIN—Liquaemin®
Anticoagulant. White powder obtained from livers or lungs of cattle, usually the sodium salt.
Absorption: Not absorbed from G. I. tract.
Actions and Uses: Anticoagulant used to prevent thromboses and blood clotting in transfusions. Effects develop quickly.
Warnings: May cause chill. Overdosage may cause serious hemorrhage. Clotting time must be carefuly followed.
Administration: Intravenous and intramuscular.
Preparations: Vial, solution containing 10 mg. per cc.
Dose: 50 mg. every 4 hours or 100 to 200 mg. in a slowly administered infusion.

HEPTABARBITAL—Medomin®
Barbiturate, hypnotic. A barbiturate with moderately rapid curve of action, but with no special superiority over others in the group. See Barbiturates.
Preparations: Tablets rather than capsules which are usual for barbiturates; in several sizes, 50 mg. (pink), 100 mg. (yellow) and 200 mg. (white).
Dose: Of the order of 200-400 mg. orally for hypnosis, 50-100 mg. for sedation.

HEROIN
A morphine derivative with high potential for addiction; no longer legally available for any purpose in this country. Commonly used by addicts.

HETRAZAN®, see Diethylcarbamazine

HEXACHLOROPHENE
—Gamophen®, Hex-O-San®, pHisoHex®, Surgi-Cen®
A phenol antiseptic used mainly in

surgical soaps in from about 0.5 to 2.5% concentration.

HEXAMETHONIUM—Bistrium®, Esomid®, Methium®
Hypotensive.
Actions and Uses: Autonomic ganglionic blocking agent. Has an action described as "medical sympathectomy." Produces a marked reduction of blood pressure in most patients with essential arterial hypertension. Reported to prolong life in malignant hypertension and materially alter the progress of the disease. Its use is definitely waning.
Warnings: Very potent drug. Must be administered under careful medical supervision. Paralytic ileus reported.
Administration: Oral, subcutaneous.
Preparations: Tablet, 250 mg. Vial, multi-dose, 25 mg. per cc.
Dose: Varies with individual patient response.

HEXAVITAMINS
Vitamin. A mixture containing 5000 units vitamin A, 400 Units vitamin D, 75 mg. abscorbic acid, 2 mg. thiamine hydrochloride, 3 mg. riboflavin, and 20 mg. nicotinamide.
Actions and Uses: As a prophylactic, a supplement to diets which may be deficient in vitamins so as to insure the proper daily vitamin intake.
Administration: Oral.
Preparations: Capsule, tablet.
Dose: Each tablet or capsule contains approximately the adult daily requirement.

HEXESTROL
Synthetic estrogen.
Actions and Uses: Much the same as diethylstilbestrol, which see.

HEXETHAL—Ortal®
One of the rapid acting barbiturates, which see.

HEXETIDINE—Sterisil®
Antiseptic. New agent used mainly as vaginal antiseptic. Action said to be especially prolonged. Claimed to be highly effective against *Trichomonas* and *He-*

mophilus Vaginalis. Available in tubes with applicators.

HEXOBARBITAL—Evipal®
Hypnotic. The sodium salt, a white powder with bitter taste soluble in water. *Actions and Uses:* One of the very rapidly acting barbiturate drugs. Used for general anesthesia of brief duration. *Warnings:* Rapid injection may induce extreme fall in blood pressure. Although recovery is relatively rapid patient may not recover completely for a much longer period and, therefore, requires observation.
Administration: Intravenous.
Preparations: Ampule containing 1 Gm. *Dose:* 2 to 4 cc. of a 10 percent solution to induce anesthesia, with increments of 1 or 2 cc. as required.
Antidote: Picrotoxin.

HEXOCYCLIUM—Tral®
Anticholinergic. Still another of this series. Superiority over others now in use to be established by long clinical trial. Available in 25 mg. tablets.

HEX-O-SAN®, see Hexachlorophene

HEXYLCAINE—Cyclaine®
Local anesthetic, which see. Available in 1·5% solutions.

HEXYLRESORCINOL
Vermifuge. White crystals, slightly soluble in water.
Actions and Uses: Topical antiseptic and anthelmintic. Used for treatment of roundworm, hookworm, whipworm and tapeworm infestations. Less toxic than aspidium and carbon tetrachloride. *Warnings:* Highly irritant to the skin, mucous membranes and respiratory tract. Pills should be well coated and swallowed without chewing.
Administration: Oral, topical.
Preparations: Pill, coated with gelatin and containing 0.1 and 0.2 Gm. Solution. *Dose:* 1.0 Gm.

HIPPURAN®, see Iodohippurate

HISTADYL®, see Methapyrilene

HISTALOG®, see Betazole

HISTAMINE
Gastric stimulant, diagnostic material, rubefacient.
Colorless crystals, soluble in water. *Actions and Uses:* Stimulates the secretion of hydrochloric acid by the stomach and used as a test for gastric activity. Said to be of value in treatment of Menière's syndrome and multiple sclerosis.
Warnings: Causes fall in blood pressure and overdosage may cause vasomotor collapse or shock. Symptoms include headache, dizziness, asthmatic attacks. *Administration:* Intramuscular, subcutaneous, also by iontophoresis for local vascular effects.
Preparations: Ampule, sterile solution, 1.0 mg. per cc.
Dose: 0.3–0.5 mg.

HISTIONEX®, see Phenyltoloxamine

HOLOCAINE®, see Phenacaine

HOMATROPINE—Mesopin®, Novatrin®
Mydriatic, anticholinergic. White crystals or powder, soluble in water, usually the hydrochloride.
Absorption: Absorbed from conjunctival surface of the eye.
Actions and Uses: Paralyzes parasympathetic nerve terminations and produces dilatation of the pupil of the eye. Actions, same as of atropine, but weaker and less persistent. Used for effects on G. I. tract as a substitute for atropine. *Warnings:* Although less liable to cause acute glaucoma than atropine, same precautions are to be oberved as with atropine.
Administration: Topical in the eye, oral. *Preparations:* Ophthalmic, discs, solution, 1–2%. Tablet, 2.5 mg. in form of the methylbromide for G. I. effects. *Dose:* Eye, about 1.5 mg. Oral 2.5–5 mg. 2–3 times daily.

HORMESTERAL®, see Estrogenic Substances, Conjugated

HORMONES
Adrenocorticotropic hormone, Anti-inflam-

matory, Androgens, Chorionic gonadotropin, Corticotropin, Cortisone, Desoxycorticosterone, Epinephrine, Estrogens, Hydrocortisone, Insulins, Parathyroid, Oxytocin, Posterior Pituitary, Progesterone, Relaxin, Testosterone, Thyroid, Vasopressin.

HYALURONIDASE — Alidase®, Diffusin®, Enzodase®, Hyazyme®, Wydase®

Spreading agent.

Actions and Uses: This is an enzyme which hydrolyzes the cement material of connective tissues and facilitates the absorption of fluids which are injected subcutaneously. Thus, the rate of absorption of clyses can be accelerated, and the rate of absorption of drugs injected subcutaneously may also be hastened. This is of great practical importance in cases in which the intravenous route may not be used for one reason or another, and yet rapid absorption is essential. Large hypodermoclyses may be more acceptable because of less discomfort when this material is used. The material is generally injected in the same syringe or in the first part of the material injected by clysis.

Warnings: Store in refrigerator. Dissolve just before using. When injecting toxic drugs, this material may hasten the rate of absorption to such an extent that toxic reaction may result.

Preparations: Vial, containing 250 viscosity units and sodium chloride. 1 cc. of injection fluid is added just prior to using. This makes an isotonic solution.

Dose: 250 viscosity units..

HYAZYME®, see Hyaluronidase

HYDELTRA®, see Prednisolone

HYDRABAMINE PENICILLIN G— Compocillin®

Another one of the long-acting forms of penicillin, which see.

HYDRALAZINE—Apresoline®

Hypotensive. Pale yellow to white crystalline material, slightly soluble in water.

Actions and Uses: Used in hypertension persisting or recurring after sympathec-

tomy, essential and early malignant hypertension, acute glomerulonephritis and certain types of toxemias of pregnancy. Mode of action unknown.

Warnings: May produce tachycardia, palpitation, dizziness, weakness, mild to severe headache, nausea and vomiting, postural hypotension, numbness and tingling of the extremities, flushing, varying degrees of nasal congestion, lacrimation, conjunctival inflammation. As therapy is continued, these untoward effects generally subside. Use with extreme caution in patients having coronary artery disease, advanced renal damage and existing or incipient cerebral accidents. Check patient's blood pressure frequently, especially after parenteral administration. Collagen disease has been reported due to its use. It may be desirable to initiate treatment parenterally in the hospitalized patient, shifting to oral therapy within 24-48 hours.

Administration: Oral, intravenous, intramuscular.

Preparations: Tablet, 25 mg., 50 mg. Vial, 10 cc., containing 20 mg. per cc.

Dose: Adjusted to the individual patient's response.

HYDRIODIC ACID

Iodide. Colorless or yellow liquid.

Actions and Uses: As a source of iodine in the treatment of thyroid gland disease. Also as an expectorant. No advantages over other iodine sources.

Warnings: Same disadvantages as other iodides. Skin eruptions.

Administration: Oral, well diluted with water.

Preparations: Syrup.

Dose: 4-8 cc. of the syrup.

HYDRIONIC®, see Glutamic Acid Hydrochloride

HYDROCHLORIC ACID

Digestive. Colorless, irritant fluid with irritant fumes.

Actions and Uses: Normally, the stomach secretes large quantities of dilute hydrochloric acid. This material is essential to proper digestive processes, although it causes considerable pain in

patient with peptic ulcer. In pernicious anemia and other conditions in which gastric acidity is markedly reduced or deficient, the oral administration of the acid is useful.
Warnings: High concentrations are irritant. Acid may erode the teeth and should be taken through a tube and in well diluted solutions.
Administration: Oral.
Preparations: Dilute hydrochloric acid (25%), further diluted with water.
Dose: 1–5 cc. of the dilute hydrochloric acid.
Antidote: Alkali, sodium bicarbonate.

HYDROCORTAMATE—
Magnacort®
Anti-inflammatory hormone, antipruritic.
Used topically in 0.5% ointment base.

HYDROCORTISONE—Cortef®, Cortril®, Hydrocortone®, Solu-Cortef®
Hormone. White crystalline powder, slightly soluble in water. Available as acetate, butylacetate, cyclopentyl propionate, and succinate.
Actions and Uses: Distinct compound and differing from cortisone, it is one of the hormonal substances isolated from extracts of the adrenal cortex and has been synthesized from a bile steroid. Injected intra-articularly, it produces local relief in joints chosen for treatment and is without generalized systemic effects. Used in treatment of rheumatoid and osteoarthritic joints.
Warnings: Should not be used in specific infectious arthritis, such as tuberculous or gonococcal. Do not dilute or mix with other substances.
Administration: Intra-articular, oral, topical.
Preparations: Vial, 5 cc. containing 25 mg. per cc. Tablets, 5, 10, 20 mg. Ointment, 1.0, 2.5%. Suspension, 0.5, 2.5%.
Dose: 10-25 mg. for parenteral or oral administration, 0.5 to 2.5% for topical application.

HYDROCORTONE®, see Hydrocortisone

HYDRODEXTRAN—Hydrox®
Plasma expander. A Dextran derivative whose advantages remain to be established.

HYDROGEN DIOXIDE, see Hydrogen Peroxide

HYDROGEN PEROXIDE— Hydrogen Dioxide
Antiseptic. A solution containing about 3% hydrogen peroxide, foams on touching skin or mucous membranes.
Actions and Uses: A mildly antibacterial material, which by its bubbling action appears to have a mechanical cleansing action as well. Not a potent or important antiseptic.
Warnings: May be irritating to mucous membranes. If solution does not foam, it is probably inert. Unstable. Do not use if the solution is old.
Administration: Topical.
Preparations: Solution, 3%.
Dose: Topical, 3% solution.

HYDROPHILIC OINTMENT
Base for ointment medication.
Actions and Uses: A white ointment base into which fatty or oil ingredients may be mixed, and which is readily washed with water. Usually used as base for skin medicaments.
Warnings: Store in cool place.

HYDROPHILIC PETROLATUM
Base.
Actions and Uses: A mixture of petrolatum containing wool fat. Usually used as a base when water soluble materials are mixed in an ointment. Facilitates penetration of ointment medicaments into hair follicles and pores.
Warnings: Store in cool place.

HYDROUS WOOL FAT, see Wool Fat

HYDROX®, see Hydrodextran

HYDROXYAMPHETAMINE— Paredrine®
Adrenergic and decongestant. White crystals, soluble in water, usually the hydrobromide.
Actions and Uses: Actions typical of

adrenergic drugs but the central effects are far less prominent than peripheral effects; nasal decongestion, mydriasis and cycloplegia.

Warnings: Repeated use may irritate nasal mucous membranes.

Administration: Topical.

Preparations: Solution, 1%.

Dose: Amount used depends on indications.

HYDROXYCHLOROQUINE— Plaquenil®

Antimalarial. Also recommended for the treatment of light-sensitive diseases and lupus erythematosus. Available in 200 mg. tablets.

HYDROXYDIONE—Viadril®

Anesthetic. Steroidal material which is used as intravenous anesthetic. Position as anesthetic remains to be established. Available in 0.5 Gm. vials.

HYDROXYPROGESTERONE— Delalutin®

Hormone. Progesterone derivative, which see. Recommended for habitual and threatened abortion.

HYDROXYZINE—Atarax®

Tranquilizer. New antihistamine drug with actions and uses much like those of Chlorpromazine, which see. Advantages over the latter and sphere of therapeutic usefulness remain to be established. Dosage ranges around 25 mg. three times a day.

HYKINONE®, see Menadione

HYOSCINE, see Scopolamine

HYOSCYAMINE—Levsin®

Anticholinergic. Much the same actions and dangers as Atropine, which see. Doses of the order of 15 mg. orally.

HYOSCYAMUS—Henbane

Antispasmodic, anticholinergic. Grayish-green powder.

Actions and Uses: Similar to belladonna, but less potent. Used in treatment of paralysis agitans, and as a depressant, but is not as effective as scopolamine. Largely falling into disuse.

Warnings: Overdosage may cause depres-sion, confusion, delirium, temperature elevation.

Administration: Oral.

Preparations: Extract, fluidextract, tincture.

Dose: Equivalent of 0.2 Gm. of the powdered hyoscyamus.

HYPAQUE®, see Diatrizoate

HYPHYLLINE—Neothylline® Xanthine derivative, which see.

HYPO, see Sodium Thiosulfate

HYPOCHLORITE SOLUTION, see Sodium Hypochlorite

HYPOTENSIVE AGENTS Central nervous system depressants, Chlorisondamine, Cryptenamine, Hexamethonium, Hydralazine, Mecamylamine, Pentolinium, Rauwolfia derivatives, Thiocyanates, Veratrum derivatives.

HYPROTIGEN®, see Amino Acid Preparations

HYTAKEROL®, see Dihydrotachysterol

I

I[131], see Radioiodine

ICHTHAMMOL—Ichthyol®

Skin antiseptic. Dark brown to black viscous fluid with characteristic odor. Miscible with water and oils.

Actions and Uses: Mild skin antiseptic used in dermatologic ointments, chiefly in cases of acne and furuncles. Not dependable.

Warnings: Stains linens. Store in cool place.

Administration: Topical. Never internally.

Preparations: Ointment.

Dose: Concentration, 10%.

ICHTHYOL®, see Ichthammol

ILETIN®, see Insulin

ILIDAR®, see Azapetine

ILOTYCIN®, see Erythromycin

IMFERON®, see Iron-Dextran

INDIGO CARMINE, see Sodium Indigotindisulfonate

INH®, see Isoniazid

**INOSITOL HEXANITRATE—
Tolanate®**
Nitrite. One of the so-called long-acting nitrite drugs. Dosage of the order of 10 mg. See Nitrites.

INSULIN—Iletin®
Hormone. Obtained from pancreas of cattle.
Actions and Uses: The natural hormone is intimately concerned with the utilization of carbohydrate after absorption into the bloodstream. Used in treatment of diabetes and other situations in which stimulation of carbohydrate metabolism is indicated. Used as convulsant in certain psychiatric conditions.
Warnings: Overdose or unusual exertion may result in insulin reaction. Symptoms include: nervousness, weakness, insomnia, diaphoresis, coma, convulsion. Store in refrigerator. Always examine label for expiration date and unitage of solution.
Administration: Subcutaneous, intravenous.
Preparations: Crystalline (regular), crystalline zinc, globin zinc, Isophane (NPH®, a mixture of insulin, protamine and zinc), protamine zinc. These preparations differ in rate of absorption from site of injection, all the others being more slowly absorbed than the crystalline insulin, and the latter is less commonly used than the others for that reason. Unitage of insulin varies and is indicated on bottle. See Insulin Preparations.
Orally effective insulin substitutes: These are now under investigation but utility in clinical diabetes remains to be established.
Dose: Depends on acuteness of condition, seriousness of diabetes and type of insulin used.
Antidote: Carbohydrate (lump of sugar, orange juice, intravenous dextrose).
Insulin color codes: Color of wrapper distinguishes the type and concentration of insulin as follows. Yellow, 20 U.S.P. Units per cc. Red, 40 U.S.P. Units per

cc. Green, 80 U.S.P. Units per cc. Orange, 100 U.S.P. Units per cc.
Gray: Indicates that crystalline insulin is present. Blue and gray, or blue, gray and yellow: 20 U.S.P. Units crystalline per cc. Red and gray: 40 U.S.P. Units crystalline insulin per cc. Green and gray: 80 U.S.P. Units crystalline insulin per cc.
White: Indicates that protamine zinc insulin is present. Red and white: 40 U.S.P. Units protamine zinc insulin per cc. Green and white: 80 U.S.P. Units protamine zinc insulin per cc.
Brown: Indicates that globin insulin with zinc is present. Red and brown: 40 U.S.P. Units globin insulin with zinc per cc. Green and brown: 80 U.S.P. Units globin insulin with zinc per cc.

INTOCOSTRIN®, see Chondodendron Tomentosum Extract

INVERSINE®, see Mecamylamine

INVERT SUGAR—Travert®
A dextrose substitute consisting of a mixture of dextrose and fructose formed by the inversion of sucrose. See Dextrose.

IODEIKON®, see Iodophthalein

IODIDES
This includes a large list of drugs which contain (1) iodine as such, (2) salts of iodine or iodides and (3) iodized drugs used largely for x-ray visualization of the lungs, gall-bladder, genito-urinary tract, spinal canal and in angiocardiography. The most common uses for the first two groups are as antiseptics and antiluetic agents although there are many other minor uses.
Allergic reactions to iodine compounds, especially skin reactions, are relatively common. Usually these can be treated by the discontinuation of the drug. Large doses of iodine can cause severe intestinal irritation, coma and death.

**IODINATED POPPYSEED OIL—
Ethiodol®**
Diagnostic. Radio-opaque iodide.

IODINE
Antiseptic. Dark metallic plates, slightly

soluble in water (more soluble when solution contains potassium or sodium iodide). Soluble in alcohol.
Actions and Uses: One of the most dependable and least expensive skin antiseptics. Commonly used for application to small cuts and bruises. Use in preparation of skin for surgery is decreasing because of local reactions. Used internally for treatment of goiter.
Warnings: Extensive application in hypersensitive patients may cause serious skin burns. Antiseptic action requires many minutes wait. After iodine dries on skin it should be removed with 70% alcohol.
Administration: Topical, oral.
Preparations: Tincture, 2, 3, 5, 7%. Lugol's solution, 5%. Talbot's solution, iodine 10%, zinc iodide, glycerine, water.
Dose: Depends on indications.
Antidote: If taken internally, give milk or eggs and evacuate stomach.

IODIPAMIDE—Cholografin®
Diagnostic. Radio-opaque iodide used for x-ray visualization of the gallbladder. Available as sodium salt and the methylglucamine. Usual dose is about 8 Gm.

IODIZED OIL—Lipiodol®
Diagnostic. A vegetable oil containing about 40% iodine in organic form.
Actions and Uses: Since it is opaque to x-ray, it is used for diagnosis as a contrast medium. The iodine may be absorbed after swallowing, and it is largely replaced by other types of contrast media.

IODOALPHIONIC ACID—
Priodax®
Diagnostic. White or yellowish powder, insoluble in water. Iodide.
Absorption: From G. I tract.
Actions and Uses: Excreted into gallbladder. Since it is opaque to x-ray, it is used for x-ray diagnosis of gallbladder disease.
Warnings: Contraindicated with cases of acute nephritis, uremia and acute G. I. disorders. May cause vomiting, diarrhea, headache, painful urination, itching, weakness.

Administration: Oral.
Preparations: Tablet, 0.5 Gm.
Dose: A schedule of dosage to be strictly followed is usually supplied by roentgenologist. Usually about 6 tablets are taken the evening before x-ray.

IODOCHLORHYDROXYQUIN—
Entero-Vioform®, Vioform®
Antiseptic. Brownish yellow powder, insoluble in water. Iodide.
Actions and Uses: An odorless substitute for iodoform. Used largely for treatment of trichomonas vaginalis and amebiasis.
Warnings: Same as other iodides.
Administration: Topical, oral.
Preparations: Powder, ointment, paste, lotion. Tablet, 0.25 Gm.
Dose: Internal, 0.75 Gm. daily. External, concentration 2–3%.

IDOCHLOROL®, see Chloriodized Oil

IODOFORM
Antiseptic. Yellowish powder with characteristic odor, insoluble in water. Iodide.
Actions and Uses: Dusting powder to promote healing and as a mild antiseptic.
Warnings: Same as other iodides.
Administration: Topical.
Preparations: Powder.
Dose: As indicated.

IODOHIPPURATE SODIUM—
Hippuran®
Diagnostic. White powder.
Actions and Uses: Radio-opaque iodide used in retrograde pyelography.
Administration: Into urethra, bladder or ureters.
Preparations: Jelly.
Dose: Concentration, 16%.

IODOMETHAMATE—Neo-Iopax®
Diagnostic. White powder, soluble in water.
Actions and Uses: Radio-opaque iodide excreted by kidney and used in intravenous pyelography, also in retrograde pyelography.
Warnings: Contraindicated in patients with reduced kidney or liver function.

Administration: Intravenous, intraurethral.
Preparations: Ampule, 50 and 75% solutions, 10, 20, 30, 50 cc.
Dose: 10-15 Gm.

IODOPHTHALEIN
—Iodeikon®

Diagnostic. Blue-violet powder, soluble in water. Salty taste. Radiopaque iodide.
Actions and Uses: Absorbed when given orally and excreted into gall-bladder. Used for x-ray examination of gall-bladder. Largely replaced by newer contrast media.
Warnings: Same as other iodine containing contrast media.
Administration: Oral, intravenous.
Preparations: Capsule, 0.5 Gm. Solution.
Dose: Oral, 0.5 Gm. per 10 Kg. of body weight, should not exceed 3.5 Gm. Intravenous, 0.3 Gm. per 10 Kg. of body weight.

IODOPYRACET—Diodrast®

Diagnostic. A solution which is clear and colorless. Radiopaque iodide.
Actions and Uses: Rapidly excreted by the kidney and, since it is opaque to x-ray, is used for diagnostic x-ray examination of kidneys and urinary tract. Also used, after intravenous injection, for angiocardiography before it is eliminated from the bloodstream.
Warnings: Sensitive patients may have severe fall in blood pressure. Solutions deteriorate rapidly in sunlight, therefore, protect from light. Do not use unclear solutions. Epinephrine solution should be on hand when injections are made. Extravasation outside of the vein causes painful reaction. Inject carefully. Precede with conjunctival test.
Administration: Intravenous.
Preparations: Conjunctival test solution. Ampule, sterile solution, 35%, 70%.
Dose: Adult urography, 20 cc. of 35% solution. Angiocardiography, determined by examination.
Antidote: Epinephrine for hypotensive reactions.

IOPANOIC ACID—Telapaque®

Diagnostic. Cream colored powder containing iodine, insoluble in water. Iodide.
Actions and Uses: Eliminated into gall-bladder and, therefore, used in x-ray diagnosis of gall-bladder disease.
Warnings: Much the same as other radio-opaque materials of this type; nausea, diarrhea, dysuria. Do not give in cases with complete obstruction of common bile duct, nephritis or uremia.
Administration: Oral. Patient must be carefully instructed about meal.
Preparations: Tablet, 0.5 Gm.
Dose: 5–6 Gm.

IOPHENDYLATE—Pantopaque®

Diagnostic agent. A fatty material, pale yellow, odorless, viscous, not readily soluble in water.
Actions and Uses: For visualization of the subarachnoid space of the central nervous system, especially. Opaque to x-ray.
Warnings: Contraindicated whenever lumbar puncture is contraindicated.
Administration: Intrathecal.
Preparations: Ampule, containing about 3 cc.
Dose: 2-5 cc.

IOPHENOXIC ACID—Teridax®

Diagnostic. Radio-opaque iodide used for x-ray visualization of the gallbladder. Dosage ranges around 50 mg. per kg. of body weight, normally.

IOTHIOURACIL—Itrumil®

Thiouracil derivative. Another of this series of drugs with similar properties but reported to have special advantages because it contains iodine. Such claims remain to be substantiated. See Thiouracil Derivatives.

IPECAC

Emetic. Pale brown powder.
Actions and Uses: An intense nauseant used as expectorant and emetic. Formerly used in amebic dysentery, but has been replaced by more potent modern drugs such as emetine, chiniofon, etc. Emesis produces vagal tone which may be useful in treatment of cardiac arrhythmias.
Warnings: May cause violent emesis.
Administration: Oral.

Preparations: Powder, fluidextract, syrup, tincture.
Dose: 0.5 cc. of fluidextract or its equivalent.

IPRAL®, see Probarbital

IPRONIAZID—Marsilid®

Nervous system stimulant. Introduced for the treatment of tuberculosis, this drug has proved to be an excitant and is now widely used as such. Its precise position as a symptomatic agent of this type remains to be established with clinical experience. Available in 10, 25 and 50 mg. tablets.

IRON

Iron compounds are one of the oldest and safest groups of drugs used in rational medicine. They are used almost exclusively in treatment of so-called iron-deficiency anemias to provide a source of iron for the formation of hemoglobin. The iron compounds are of little value in the treatment of anemias due to active infectious processes and primary anemias.

In general, any iron salt, or even metallic iron itself, may be used in the treatment of the iron-deficiency anemias. Iron salts are slowly and poorly absorbed from G.I. tract. For that reason, small doses are without much effect and relatively large doses of iron must be used. Iron may be given by parenteral injection but the amount necessary is so large that, generally, this method of administration is impractical and painful. The oral route is route of choice.

The chief difficulty with iron salts, is the tendency to cause G. I. distress, nausea, loss of appetite and diarrhea. In many instances this can be overcome by administering the iron immediately after meals. In some instances the patient can tolerate only certain iron compounds, and it is well to look for these when patients have trouble with their iron medication. The ferrous salts of iron are preferred to the ferric salts since they seem to be somewhat more effective and also less irritant. Arsenical iron compounds (cacodylates) are not frequently used today.

All iron compounds tend to turn stools dark green or black; patients should be warned of this.

Iron compounds: Ferric ammonium citrate, Ferric cacodylate, Ferric chloride, Ferric glycerophosphate, Ferric hypophosphite, Ferric oxide, Ferric phosphate, Ferric subsulfate, Ferrous carbonate, Ferrous gluconate, Ferrous iodide, Ferrous sulfate, Iron Glycamine.

IRON BILE SALTS—Bilron®, see Ox Bile Extract

IRON-DEXTRAN—Imferon®

Hematinic. Evidence is presented that this drug is effective by intramuscular injection. Available in 50 mg. ampules.

IRON GLUCONATE, see Ferrous Gluconate

IRON GLYCAMINE—Ferronord®

Hematinic. Iron salt, which see, said to be better than ordinarily absorbed, less irritant to the G.I. tract. Dosage of the order of 125 mg. Unless this material is exceptionally well absorbed, this is an exceedingly small dose.

IRON SULFATE, see Ferrous Sulfate

I-SEDRINE®, see Ephedrine

ISOBORNYL THIOCYANOACE-TATE—Bornate®

Parasiticide. Yellow oily liquid, not miscible with water.
Actions and Uses: For treatment of pediculosis.
Warnings: Do not apply near eyes or mucous membranes.
Administration: Topical.
Preparations: Emulsion, 5%.
Dose: 5% emulsion.

ISODINE®, see Povidone-Iodine

ISOFLUROPHATE—DFP, Floropryl®

Cholinergic. Usually in dilute solution.
Actions and Uses: Produces intense cholinergic effects by preventing destruction of acetylcholine formed in body; local application in eye causes miosis, systemic action, intense intestinal activity and salivation.

Warnings: Potent drug which may cause serious poisoning in overdose; toxic effects may include nausea, vomiting, diarrhea, hypotension, bradycardia, and asthmatic attacks.
Administration: Usually topical in eye.
Preparations: Ophthalmic solution, 0.1% in peanut oil.
Dose: A few drops of above solution in eye.
Antidote: Atropine.

ISO-IODEIKON®, see Phentetiothalein

ISOMETHEPTENE—Octin®
Antispasmodic. A sympathetic-like substance which produces relaxation by sympathetic stimulation rather than the anticholinergic action of most other antispasmodics. Produces also, therefore, some vasoconstriction, cardiac stimulation, and increase in blood pressure. Therapeutic status remains to be established. Administered orally and intramuscularly. Usual dosage is of the order of 50 to 100 mg.

ISONIAZID—Isonicotinic Acid Hydrazide, Armazide®, Cotinazin® Dinacrin®, Ditubin®, INH®, Niadrin®, Niconyl®, Nicozide®, Nydrazid®, Pyrizidin®, Rimifon®, Tisin®, Tyvid®, Zinadon®
Antitubercular.
Absorption: Rapidly absorbed from G. I. tract with high levels found within 2 hours in the plasma, cerebrospinal fluid and other body fluids.
Actions and Uses: Used in the emergency treatment of patients with tuberculosis, usually in combination with other antitubercular drugs or antibiotics. Has been found to have a marked effect in reducing fever and in promoting appetite, body weight and strength, with significant reduction in cough and expectoration.
Warnings: There is evidence that there is an emergence of resistant strains after contact with the drug for varying periods of time. Promiscuous or indiscriminate use may result in lack of therapeutic efficacy at the time when the patient may need the drug for emergency use.

Administration: Oral.
Preparations: Tablet, 50 mg., 100 mg.
Dose: 2-4 mg. per Kg. of body weight daily in divided doses, should not exceed 150-200 mg. per day.

ISONICOTINIC ACID HYDRAZIDE, see Isoniazid

ISONORIN®, see Isoproterenol

ISO-PAR®, see Coparaffinate

ISOPHANE INSULIN—NPH Insulin
Modified neutral protamine zinc insulin. See Insulin.

ISOPHRIN®, see Phenylephrine

ISOPROPYL ALCOHOL
Local antiseptic and solvent. Clear colorless fluid with characteristic odor.
Actions and Uses: Mild skin antiseptic, which is commonly found in rubbing alcohols sold on the open market instead of ethyl alcohol. The isopropyl alcohol so sold, is not particularly dependable as a skin disinfectant.
Warnings: Exceedingly toxic, if taken by mouth. Store in cool place.
Administration: Topical.
Preparations: Solution, 70% by weight.
Dose: Topical, concentration of 70%.

ISOPROPYLARTERENOL, see Isoproterenol

ISOPROTERENOL—Aludrine®, Isonorin®, Isuprel®, Norisodrine®
Adrenergic. Bitter crystals; the hydrochloride and sulfate salts are freely soluble in water.
Actions and Uses: Related to epinephrine but with much less effect on blood pressure; large doses may even produce a fall. Has pronounced direct effect on heart to accelerate it. Is potent antiallergic and antiasthmatic. Used principally in allergic asthma to relieve these attacks (without other epinephrine effects) and in Stokes-Adams attacks of heart block.
Administration: Inhalation, sublingual.
Preparations: Inhalant solution, 1:200,

1:100. Tablet, 10, 15 mg. Powder (inhalant), 10, 25%.
Warnings: May produce extreme tachycardia, with precordial distress, shock and electrocardiographic changes. It is to be used with caution, therefore, in patients with heart disease, especially after myocardial occlusion.
Dose: Varies with indication.

ISUPREL®, see Isoproterenol

ITRUMIL®, see Iothiouracil

J

JALAP
Cathartic. Light brown powder.
Actions and Uses: Drastic cathartic.
Warnings: In common with all cathartics, continued use tends toward habituation.
Administration: Oral.
Preparations: Powder and resin.
Dose: Powder, 1.0 Gm. Resin, 0.1 Gm.

JAMESTOWN WEED, see Stramonium

JIMSON WEED, see Stramonium

JUNIPER TAR—Cade Oil
Parasiticide. A dark brown liquid with tarry odor. To be distinguished from juniper derived from the berry of another plant, which is used as a flavor.
Actions and Uses: Skin irritant and stimulant. Used in psoriasis and chronic eczema, and a parasiticide against scabies and favus.
Warnings: Store in cool place.
Administration: Topical.
Preparations: Ointment.
Dose: Concentration, 1–10%.

K

KAOLIN
Absorbent. Whitish clayey powder, insoluble in water.
Absorption: Not absorbed from G. I. tract.
Actions and Uses: Acts as a physical absorbent. Used to absorb moisture and toxins, externally in skin preparations and internally, for the same action in the intestine.
Warnings: For greatest effectiveness, used in finely divided form. Mix well and discard lumps.
Administration: Topical, oral.
Preparations: Powder and cataplasm.
Dose: Oral, 15–60 Gm. External, as indicated.

KATONIUM®, see Styronate Resins

KEMADRIN®, see Procyclidine

KERATOLYTIC AGENTS
Chrysarobin, Salicylic acid.

KHELISEM®, see Visammin

KHELLIN, see Visammin

KINAVOSYL®, see Mephenesin

KONOGEN®, see Estrogenic Substances, Conjugated

KWELL®, see Benzene Hexachloride, Gamma

L

LABARRAQUE'S SOLUTION, see Sodium Hypochlorite

LACTATED RINGER'S SOLUTION—Hartmann's Solution
Parenteral fluid. Clear, colorless solution when diluted, containing physiologic concentrations of sodium lactate, sodium, potassium and calcium chloride and water.
Actions and Uses: Used in the management of acidosis associated with dehydration and loss of electrolyte.
Warnings: Concentrates must be accurately diluted.
Administration: Intravenous, subcutaneous.
Preparations: Ampule, 20 cc. to be diluted in 500 cc.
Dose: Variable, determined by individual patient response.

LACTOFLAVIN, see Riboflavin

LACTOSE—Milk Sugar
Nutritional, vehicle.
A white powder with faint sweet taste.

Absorption: Well absorbed from G. I. tract.
Actions and Uses: As a food, usually in infant formulas. Less sweet than cane sugar, therefore better tolerated in large doses. Has slight laxative action.
Warnings: Gas formation common after large amounts.
Administration: Oral.
Preparations: Powder. Tablet, see Placebo.
Dose: 30–60 Gm. daily.

LANATOSIDE C—Cedilanid®
Purified digitalis material. White powder, insoluble in water.
Absorption: Moderately well absorbed from G. I. tract.
Actions and Uses: See digitalis. In general, effects come on somewhat more rapidly than after digitalis leaf or digitoxin. Excreted more rapidly than the latter. Very much like digoxin in all its properties.
Warnings: Same as for all forms of digitalis.
Administration: Oral, intramuscular, intravenous.
Preparations: Tablet and ampule.
Dose: Oral, 0.5 mg. Parenteral, 0.5 mg.
Antidote: None.

LANOLIN, see Wool Fat

LANOXIN®, see Digoxin

LASSAR'S PASTE, see Zinc Oxide

LAUDANUM, see Opium

LAUGHING GAS, see Nitrous Oxide

LAURON®, see Aurothioglycanide

LAXATIVES, see Cathartics

LEAD ACETATE—Sugar of Lead
Astringent. Colorless crystals, soluble in water.
Actions and Uses: Astringent for lotions. Largely replaced by other drugs because of danger of toxicity.
Warnings: Highly toxic internally.
Administration: Topical.
Preparations: Lead and opium wash.
Dose: Concentration, 1% solution.
Antidote: Edathamil.

LEAD SUBACETATE
Much the same as lead acetate.

LECITHIN COMPOUND
Cholegogue. Thick, yellow fluid with pleasant flavor.
Actions and Uses: Used in conjunction with gall-bladder x-rays to stimulate emptying of the gall-bladder.
Warnings: Store in cool place. Do not give in complete obstruction of common bile duct.
Administration: Oral.
Preparations: Mixture containing lecithin, glycerin, egg yolk.
Dose: 30 Gm.

LEMON OIL
Flavoring agent.

LEMON PEEL
Flavoring agent.

LENIGALLOL®, see Acetpyrogall

LENTE ILETIN®, see Lente Insulin

LENTE INSULIN—Lente Iletin®
Suspension of zinc insulin crystals and amorphous insulin. See Insulin.

LESCOPINE®, see Methscopolamine

LEUKERAN®, see Chlorambucil

LEVALLORPHAN—Lorfan®
Morphine antagonist. Apparently similar in actions and uses to Nalorphine, which see.

LEVARTERENOL—Arterenol, Levophed®, Nor-Epinephrine
Adrenergic.
Actions and Uses: Potent pressor material producing rise in blood pressure by peripheral vasoconstriction. On the coronary arteries, may cause vasodilatation and therefore, have an effect in increasing coronary flow. Used in maintenance of blood pressure in acute hypotensive states, surgical and nonsurgical trauma, central vasomotor depression and hemorrhage.
Warnings: Because of potency and individual variations to pressor substances, the possibility of producing dangerously high blood pressure with overdoses always exists. It is desirable to check the

blood pressure every 2 minutes from the time the drug is started until the desired pressure is obtained, then every 5 minutes if the administration is to be continued. The rate of flow must be watched constantly and the patient should never be left unattended while receiving this drug. Contraindicated whenever cyclopropane anesthesia is used or when myocardial ischemia is suspected because of the increased possibility of ventricular fibrillation. Despite statements to the contrary, may exert a direct action on the myocardium to induce arrhythmias; should therefore be used with caution in myocardial occlusion and heart disease in general.

Administration: Intravenous.
Preparations: Ampule, 4 cc. of 1:1000 solution.
Dose: 4 cc. of 1:1000 solution added to 1000 cc. of infusion solution, blood, or plasma. Each 1 cc. of this dilution contains 4 mg. of the drug. Dosage and rate of flow determined for individual patient.

LEVO-DROMORAN®, see Levorphanol

LEVOPHED®, see Levarterenol

LEVORPHANOL—Levo-Dromoran®
Addictive analgesic. The tartrate.
Actions and Uses: Much the same as morphine. See also Racemorphan.
Warnings: Toxicity and addiction potential does not differ significantly from morphine, which see.
Administration: Oral and subcutaneous.
Preparations: Tablet, 2 mg. Ampule, 2 mg. per cc.
Dose: 2 mg.
Antidote: Nalorphine.

LEVOTHYROXINE SODIUM—Synthyroid Sodium®
Hormone. Twice as active as the racemic form, but otherwise the same as Thyroxin, which see.

LEVSIN®, see Hyoscyamine

LEVUGEN®, see Fructose

LEVULOSE, see Fructose

LICORICE POWDER, see Senna, Compound Powder

LICORICE ROOT, see Glycyrrhiza

LIDOCAINE—Xylocaine®
One of the large group of local anesthetics. See Anesthetics, local.

LIME—Calcium Oxide
Disinfectant. Hard white granules.
Actions and Uses: To disinfect excreta.

LINSEED—Flaxseed
Demulcent. Yellowish-brown powder.
Actions and Uses: Used as a demulcent and in poultices.
Warnings: Disinfect before using.
Administration: Topical. Make a thick paste of the meal with hot water, in poultices.
Preparations: Powder.
Dose: As needed.

LINSEED OIL—Flaxseed Oil
Demulcent. Oil from linseed.
Actions and Uses: As emollient oil in liniments.

LIOTHYRONINE—Cytomel®
Thyroid hormone. Said to have practical advantages over crude thyroid materials. These are yet to be clearly defined and established. Available in 5 and 25 mg. tablets.

LIPIODOL®, see Iodized Oil

LIQUAEMIN®, see Heparin

LIQUID PETROLATUM, see Petrolatum

LIQUIFIED PHENOL, see Phenol

LIQUOR ANTISEPTICUS, see Antiseptic Solution

LISSEPHEN®, see Mephenesin

LITHIUM SALTS
Warnings: A recent experience with lithium has thrown these drugs, long used only rarely, into discard. Lithium chloride was found to resemble table salt markedly in taste, and the salt was, therefore, sold widely as a salt substitute in the salt-restricted diet. Within a short period of time many of these patients suffered serious neurologic reactions and some died. It has been proven that the

75

lithium is highly toxic to the central nervous system. There is no justification for using these drugs in medicine.

LIVER

Liver, in a variety of forms, has life-saving properties for several types of primary anemia. It is to be noted that it is without any value in the iron-deficiency anemias, in which iron is effective, and it has no special virtues for normal people.

Well-cooked liver has little antianemic value, while raw or nearly raw liver is exceedingly difficult for patients to take. A list of more acceptable oral preparations has been introduced. There are also many parenteral preparations. These, supplemented with stomach preparations (which are also effective), folic acid materials and vitamin B_{12} have now entirely replaced raw liver in the treatment of primary anemia.

There are other conditions in which crude liver extracts are preferable to the highly purified, especially because of the vitamin content of the former.

Parenteral liver extracts should be injected intramuscularly, deep into the gluteal muscles.

Look for expiration date on liver preparations before using.

Liver preparations: Liver extract (dry liver extract for oral use), Liver injection (for parenteral use, contains 10 Units per cc.), Crude liver injection (contains about 1-2 Units per cc.), Liver solution (for oral use).

Liver concentrates are used for vitamin B content rather than pernicious anemia actions: Liver concentrate, Liver fraction 1, Liver fraction 2, Dried liver, Liver with stomach (oral material, 12 capsules contain 1 Unit), Powdered stomach (oral preparation).

LOBELIA

Emetic and expectorant. Infrequently used in modern medicine.

Warnings: Highly toxic with much the characteristics of nicotine.

LOBELINE—Bantron®

An old drug once used to break tobacco

habit, discarded as useless, and now revived for the same purpose.

LORFAN®, see Levallorphan

LOROTHIDOL®, see Bithionol

LOTIO ALBA, see White Lotion

LOTUSATE®, see Talbutal

LSD-25, see Lysergic Acid Diethylamide

LUCORTEUM®, see Progesterone

LUGOL'S SOLUTION, see Iodine

LUMINAL® see Phenobarbital

LUNAR CAUSTIC, see Silver Nitrate

LUNOSOL®, see Silver Chloride

LUTOCYLIN®, see Progesterone

LUTOCYLOL®, see Ethisterone

LUTREXIN®, see Lututrin

LUTROMONE®, see Progesterone

LUTUTRIN—Lutrexin®

Uterine relaxant. Ovarian extractive.

Actions and Uses: Said to relax uterus by a specific action. Therapeutic value of this drug is yet to be firmly established.

Warnings: A new drug, toxicity not yet fully determined.

Administration: Oral.

Preparations: Tablet, 1000 units.

Dose: 2000-4000 units 2-3 times daily.

LYCOPODIUM

Absorbent. Yellow powder from spores of *Lycopodium*.

Actions and Uses: Absorbent powder. Largely replaced by other materials for dusting powder. Now used chiefly as a dust to prevent pills from sticking together.

LYNORAL®, see Ethinyl Estradiol

LYSERGIC ACID DIETHYLAMIDE
—d-Lysergic Acid, Delysid®, LSD-25

Hallucinogen. This agent has recently come in for a great deal of discussion because it is hallucinogenic, i.e. its use is followed by visions and other symptoms which simulate mental disorders. It is used only in experimental studies.

M

MAGNACORT®, see Hydro-
cortamate

MAGNAMYCIN®, see Carbomycin

MAGNESIA MAGMA—
Milk of Magnesia
Antacid and laxative. A suspension of
magnesium hydroxide (8%) in water.
Actions and Uses: See Magnesium.
Warnings: See Magnesium. Shake well.
Administration: Oral.
Dose: 4–30 cc.

MAGNESIUM
Salts of magnesium are relatively non-
irritant and poorly absorbed. Given in
relatively large doses, they tend to act as
cathartics by increasing the fluid content
of the bowel.
On the other hand, when magnesium is
absorbed, it acts as a strong depressant
and can, if given parenterally, produce
depression of the brain, narcosis and
even death. The danger of absorption in
amounts sufficient to produce such effects
is present whenever large doses of magnesium salts are given over long periods
of time, especially in cases in which
there is sluggish elimination of the drug.
This danger is probably greater in the
case of the soluble salts of magnesium.
Forms of magnesium hydroxide also act
as intestinal antacids and have, therefore, the combined action of antacids
and cathartics.
Magnesium sulfate, by intramuscular injection, has been used as a central depressant and anticonvulsant, especially in
eclampsia, but because of inherent dangers this practice has largely fallen into
disuse.
Antidote. Calcium given slowly intravenously.

MAGNESIUM CARBONATE
Antacid and laxative. White odorless and
tasteless powder available in "light" and
"heavy" forms, depending on mode of
preparation. Insoluble in water.
Actions and Uses: See Magnesium.
Administration: Oral.

Preparations:. Powder.
Dose: 0.5–8 Gm.

MAGNESIUM CITRATE—
Citrate of Magnesia
Saline laxative. White crystals, powder
or granules.
Actions and Uses: Used only in the form
of a solution. Laxative.
Warnings: See Magnesium.
Administration: Oral.
Preparations: Magnesium citrate solution,
usually dispensed in citric acid, and car-
bonated, so that it effervesces.
Dose: 200–350 cc.

MAGNESIUM HYDROXIDE
Antacid and laxative. White powder with
no taste or odor. Insoluble in water.
Actions and Uses: Used mainly in milk
of magnesia. See Magnesium.
Warnings: See Magnesium.
Administration: Oral.
Preparations: Milk of magnesia solution.
Tablet.
Dose: 0.3 Gm.

MAGNESIUM OXIDE
Antacid and laxative. White bulky odor-
less and tasteless powder, available in
"light" and "heavy" forms, depending
on mode of preparation. Insoluble in
water.
Actions and Uses: See Magnesium.
Warnings: See Magnesium.
Administration: Oral.
Preparations: Powder.
Dose: 0.25–4 Gm.

MAGNESIUM PHOSPHATE
Antacid. White powder, insoluble in
water.
Actions and Uses: See Magnesium.
Warnings: See Magnesium.
Administration: Oral.
Preparations: Powder. Tablet, 0.3 and
0.5 Gm.
Dose: 1 Gm.

MAGNESIUM SULFATE—
Epsom Salts
Saline cathartic. Colorless crystals with
a bitter, salty taste.
Actions and Uses: Salt in hot soaks,
baths, etc., in inflammatory conditions.

Solutions are occasionally used for the central depressant action in convulsive and tetanic states, but this use is dangerous and limited, and in recent years has been replaced by other less dangerous drugs. Widely used as a saline cathartic. See Magnesium.
Warnings: See Magnesium.
Administration: Oral, intravenous.
Preparations: Salt. Solution, parenteral (25%).
Dose: Cathartic, 15 Gm. Depressant, 25 mg. per Kg. body weight.
Antidote: Calcium salts intravenously. Should be kept on hand for immediate use in cases in which magnesium is being used for its depressant action.

MAGNESIUM TRISILICATE
Antacid. Fine white powder, insoluble in water.
Actions and Uses: See Magnesium.
Warnings: See Magnesium.
Administration: Oral.
Preparations: Tablet, 0.3 and 0.5 Gm. Gel, with aluminum hydroxide.
Dose: 1 Gm.

MAIZE OIL, see Corn Oil
MALE FERN OLEORESIN, see Aspidium Oleoresin
MALESTRONE®, see Testosterone
MALT
Nutritional. Yellowish grains with characteristic odor and taste.
Actions and Uses: A malted form of barley, used as a food, to digest starch with its enzymes. As a vehicle and emulsifier.
Preparations: Extract, cod liver oil emulsion.
Dose: 15 Gm.

MANDELAMINE®, see Methenamine Mandelate
MANDELIC ACID
Urinary antiseptic.
Actions and Uses: Excreted into urinary tract where it acts as a potent antiseptic against many of the common causes of urinary tract infections. Now largely replaced by sulfonamides, antibiotics and mandelate salts.

MANGANESE COMPOUNDS
Actions and Uses: Used mainly as hematinics with doubtful value. In view of the much more effective drugs now available, have been largely discarded.
MANNITOL HEXANITRATE—
   Nitranitol®
Coronary artery dilator.
Actions and Uses: Mainly for relaxation of spasm of the coronary arteries in attacks of angina pectoris. Action is more slow to develop and longer-lasting than with nitroglycerine. Used also to prevent attacks. Action is much the same as that of nitroglycerine.
Warnings: May depress bone marrow.
Administration: Oral.
Preparations: Tablet, 30 mg.
Dose: 30 mg. every 4–6 hours. Use smallest dose that is effective.

MAPHARSEN®, see Oxophenarsine
MAREZINE®, see Cyclizine
MARIHUANA, see Cannabis
MARSILID®, see Iproniazid
MASENATE®, see Testosterone
MATROMYCIN®, see Oleandomycin
MEBARAL®, see Mephobarbital
MECAMYLAMINE—Inversine®
Hypotensive. Another new ganglionic blockader introduced for the treatment of hypertension. Value, advantages, and dangers remain to be established. Dosage ranges from 2.5 to 10 mg.

MECHLORETHAMINE—Nitrogen
   Mustard, Mustargen®
Anticarcinogenic.
Dry powder, usually the hydrochloride, soluble in water.
Actions and Uses: An antimitotic agent which restrains the growth of several forms of malignant tumors but does not cure them. May be especially valuable in areas in which x-ray and radium therapy are not available.
Warnings: Usually depresses bone marrow, may induce serious granulocytopenia; contact with skin, mucous membranes and eyes to be avoided.
Administration: Intravenous.

Preparations: Vial containing 10 mg. dry drug and sodium chloride, to be dissolved before using.
Dose: 0.1 mg. per Kg. body weight.

MECHOLYL®, see Methacholine

MECLIZINE—Bonamine®
A drug of the antihistamine series said to be especially useful in the prevention and treatment of nausea, vomiting and motion sickness. See Antihistaminics.

MECOSTRIN®, see Dimethyl-Tubocurarine

MEDICINAL SOFT SOAP, see Soap, Medicinal, Soft

MEDICINAL ZINC PEROXIDE, see Zinc Peroxide

MEDOMIN®, see Heptabarbital

MEDROL®, see Methylprednisolone

MELAMINE, see Triethylene Melamine

MENADIONE—Vitamin K, Hykinone®
Vitamin. Bright yellow powder, insoluble in water, but salts of which are water soluble.
Absorption: Absorbed from G. I. tract.
Actions and Uses: In hemorrhagic states due to vitamin K deficiency, low prothrombin content of the blood, liver disease, Dicumarol® (and related drugs) intoxication, obstructive jaundice, hemorrhagic disease of the newborn. Water soluble forms do not require fat or bile to assure absorption.
Administration: Oral, intramuscular, subcutaneous, intravenous.
Preparations: Capsule, 1 mg. Solution, in oil. Tablet, 1 mg. Soluble sodium bisulfite in 4 mg. capsule, sterile solution in water; 4 mg. in 1 cc. and 72 mg. in 10 cc.
Dose: 4 mg. daily for deficiency states. 72 mg. intravenously for Dicumarol® intoxication.

MENTHOL
Counterirritant and skin coolant. Clear colorless crystals with characteristic odor. Slightly soluble in water.

Actions and Uses: Counterirritant. Produces sensation of coolness of skin, both of which are used in treatment of skin conditions; mild local anesthetic action.
Warnings: Systemic action is that of central nervous system stimulant, producing convulsions and death. This may result from internal use or from topical application of very large doses over large surfaces of the skin.
Administration: Topical.
Preparations: Ointment. Guaiacol and menthol mixture. Powder, menthol and sodium bicarbonate. Lotion.
Dose: Topical, concentration of 1–10%.

MEONINE®, see Methionine

MEPACRINE®, see Quinacrine

MEPAZINE—Pacatal®
Tranquilizer. Chlorpromazine congener with much the same actions and dangers. Final position in therapy will be established only after long clinical experience. Available in 25 and 50 mg. tablets and solution for parenteral administration.

MEPERIDINE—Demerol®
Addictive analgesic. White powder, soluble in water.
Actions and Uses: Analgesic. Not as potent as morphine; about as effective as codeine. Unlike them as it relaxes rather than increases tone of intestine and smooth muscle and has no constipating action. Less euphoria produced than with morphine.
Warnings: More addicting than codeine. Addiction a real danger with continued use. Nausea and vomiting occur frequently.
Administration: Oral, intramuscular.
Preparations: Tablet, 50 mg. Sterile solution, 2 cc. ampules containing 100 mg. Vial, multidose.
Dose: 50–200 mg.
Antidote: Nalorphine.

MEPHENESIN—Daserol®, Dioloxol®, Kinavosyl®, Lissephen®, Mepherol®, Mephson®, Myanesin®, Myoten®, Myoxane®, Oranixon®, Prolax®, Sinan®, Spasmolyn®, Tolansin®, Toloxyn®,

Tolseram®, Tolserol®, Tolulexin®, Tolulox®, Tolyspaz®
Muscle relaxant. White powder, barely soluble in water, also the carbamate.
Absorption: From G. I. tract.
Actions and Uses: Has sedative action, but in addition provides relief from muscular tremor. May be used for a diagnostic test.
Warnings: May produce muscular weakness. Also may produce visual disturbances, and lack of muscular coordination.
Administration: Oral, parenteral.
Preparations: Capsule, tablet, 250 and 500 mg. Elixir, 100 mg. per cc.
Dose: 1 Gm. given 3–5 times daily.

MEPHENTERMINE—Wyamine®
One of the large series of adrenergic drugs, which see. Used especially for vasoconstrictant action.

MEPHEROL®, see Mephenesin

MEPHOBARBITAL—Mebaral®
Sedative. White crystals, barely soluble in water.
Actions and Uses: One of the long acting barbiturates, hence useful for prolonged sedation. Also useful for prevention of epileptic seizures.
Warnings: As for all barbiturates, may induce dependence; sudden withdrawal may be followed by convulsions in some patients.
Administration: Oral.
Preparations: Tablet, 0.1 and 0.2 Gm.
Dose: 0.03 to 0.2 Gm.
Antidote: Picrotoxin.

MEPHSON®, see Mephenesin

MEPHYTON®, see Phytonadione

MEPRANE®, Promethestrol

MEPROBAMATE—Equanil®, Miltown®
One of a number of new drugs introduced recently which exert central depressant action as well as a degree of muscle relaxation. These are said to be especially valuable in the treatment of anxiety states. Whereas their use is increasing, their final value remains to be established and, until then, especially

because their toxicity and potential for addiction have not been determined, they should be used with considerable circumspection. Administered orally; available as 400 mg. tablets.

MERALLURIDE—Mercuhydrin®
Mercurial diuretic. White to yellow powder, soluble in alkaline solutions.
Actions and Uses: Same as other mercurial diuretics, but somewhat less irritant than most. Therefore may be given subcutaneously as well as intramuscularly. Intravenous injections have been largely restricted to special situations because of occasional accidents. Used mainly in treatment of congestive heart failure.
Warnings: Contraindicated in acute nephritis. Continued frequent use presents danger of low-salt syndrome.
Administration: Intramuscular, subcutaneous.
Preparations: Ampule, 2 cc. of a 10% solution with theophylline. Tablet, rarely used. Suppository, rarely used.
Dose: 1-2 cc. as needed.
Antidote: Dimercaprol.

MERATRAN®, see Pipradol

MERBAK®, see Acetomeroctol

MERBROMIN—Mercurochrome®
Organic mercurial antiseptic. Green granules, soluble in water and alcohol, making a red solution with green-yellow fluorescence.
Actions and Uses: One of the less dependable mercurial antiseptics. Much less commonly used today than years ago.
Warnings: For external use only. Not especially dependable.
Administration: Topical.
Preparations: Tincture and aqueous solution.
Dose: Concentration, 2%.
Antidote: Dimercaprol.

MERCAPTOMERIN—Diucardyn®, Thiomerin®
Mercurial diuretic. White powder, soluble in water.
Actions and Uses: Same as other mercurial diuretics. Less irritant, and said

to be also less toxic, than any of the others. May be used subcutaneously.
Warnings: As for all mercurial diuretics (see Meralluride). Mercaptomerin seems especially prone to induce hypersensitivity, hence, observe carefully for local and systemic reactions. Examine solution for sediment. Store in cool place. Discard if turbid.
Administration: Subcutaneous, intramuscular, intravenous, rectal.
Preparations: Vial, 10 cc. containing powder to which 10 cc. of water is added. This solution will keep for several days if refrigerated. Good as long as clear. Suppositories, 0.5 Gm. Also available in solutions with a stabilizer.
Dose: 1–2 cc. above solution.
Antidote: Dimercaprol.

MERCAPTOPURINE—Purinethol®
Metabolic antagonist. Used in leukemia. Although it does not alter the fatal outcome of leukemia, it appears to induce remissions and to prolong life. Administered in oral doses (divided) of about 100 to 200 mg. daily.

MERCOCREOSOLS—Mercresin®
An organic mercurial antiseptic. See Mercury.
Antidote: Dimercaprol.

MERCRESIN®, see Mercocreosols

MERCUHYDRIN®, see Meralluride

MERCUMATILIN—Cumertilin®
Mercurial diuretic. The most recent of the mercurial diuretics listed.
Absorption: Absorbed from the G. I. tract and after intramuscular injection.
Actions and Uses: Much the same as other mercurial diuretics except it may be used orally as well as parenterally.
Warnings: The same as for other mercurial diuretics, which see.
Administration: Oral and intramuscular.
Preparations: Tablets, 65 mg. Ampules, 1-2 cc.
Dose: As with other mercurial diuretics.
Antidote: Dimercaprol.

MERCUPURIN®, see Mercurophylline

MERCURIAL DIURETICS
Chlormerodrin, Meralluride, Mercaptomerin, Mercumatilin, Mercurophylline, Mersalyl and Theophylline.

MERCURIC CHLORIDE, see Mercury Bichloride

MERCURIC IODIDE, RED
Antiseptic. Red powder, insoluble in water.
Actions and Uses: See Mercury.
Warnings: Danger same as with mercuric chloride.
Antidote: Dimercaprol.

MERCURIC OXIDE, YELLOW
Antiseptic. Orange-yellow powder, insoluble in water.
Actions and Uses: Used especially in eye infections.
Warnings: See Mercury. Attacks most metals. Do not use on instruments.
Administration: Topical in eye.
Preparations: Ointment.
Dose: Concentration, 1%.
Antidote: Dimercaprol.

MERCUROCHROME®, see Merbromin

MERCUROPHYLLINE—Mercuzanthin®, Mercupurin®
Organic mercurial diuretic. White powder, soluble in water.
Actions and Uses: Potent diuretic used in treatment of congestive heart failure.
Warnings: Excessive dosage may lead to low-sodium syndrome. Contraindicated in acute kidney conditions. Paravenous injection may cause local necrosis. Inject well into gluteal muscle.
Administration: Intramuscular, intravenous.
Preparations: Solution, 10% containing aminophyllin 5% in 1 and 2 cc. ampule.
Dose: 1 to 2 cc.; frequency as indicated by condition.
Antidote: Dimercaprol.

MERCUROUS CHLORIDE, MILD —Calomel
Cathartic. White powder, insoluble in water.
Actions and Uses: Fairly potent, slowly

acting cathartic. Now rarely used, although formerly quite a common drug.
Warnings: Should be followed by saline cathartic for if not completely eliminated, absorption may occur with resultant systemic mercury reactions.
Administration: Oral, topical.
Preparations: Tablet. Ointment, topically as an antisyphilitic. Mixture, with other cathartics (compound calomel pills).
Dose: Oral, 120 mg. Topical, concentration 30%.
Antidote: Dimercaprol.

MERCUROUS IODIDE, YELLOW
Antiluetic. Rarely used.

MERCURY
Mercury compounds have long been used in medicine, often with good results, sometimes with disasters. There are three groups: (1) mercurous, (2) mercuric, (3) organic mercurials.
Mercurous compounds are generally less toxic because of insolubility and poor absorption. Calomel (mercurous chloride) is the most common form, an effective and safe cathartic providing it is rapidly eliminated. In instances of delayed elimination absorption may result in systemic toxic effects.
Mercuric compounds, of which mercuric chloride is the best known, are the most dangerous mercury salts. They are absorbed rapidly, damage tissues, especially the kidneys. They are corrosive, not only to tissues, but even to metal instruments. No longer considered useful general antiseptic because of toxicity, corrosive action, and ineffectiveness against spores. These compounds are contraindicated for internal use.
Organic mercurials have reduced toxicity. Widely used for local antisepsis (Mertaphen®, Merthiolate®, etc.). In other forms, used as mercurial diuretics. Acute toxic reactions are relatively rare from these forms. Now rarely used as antisyphilitics. Metallic mercury (blue mass) used as antisyphilitic and topical parasitide.
Antidote for all mercurials: Dimercaprol.
Mercury compounds: Mercurial diuretics,

Mercurial antiseptics, Mercuric chloride, Mercuric iodide, Mercuric oxycyanide, Mercurous chloride, mild, Mercurous iodide.

MERCURY, AMMONIATED,
see Ammoniated Mercury

MERCURY BICHLORIDE—
Mercuric Chloride
Corrosive, antiseptic.
Colorless crystals, soluble in water.
Absorption: Rapidly absorbed from all mucous membranes.
Actions and Uses: Germicide, antiseptic, antisyphilitic.
Warnings: Rapidly produces irreversible kidney damage. Extremely rapidly absorbed from all mucous membranes. Use as a vaginal douche is dangerous for that reason. Rapidly corrosive to all tissues. Attacks metals. Because of its great toxicity, and danger of accidental administration, as well as because of more effective drugs, this material has little place in modern pharmacopeia, and for that reason, has been eliminated from many hospital formularies.
Preparations: Tablet, usually of distinctive shape and color.
Dose: Concentration, as antiseptic 1:1000-1:20,000. Tablets are made in such sizes that such dilutions can be made easily.
Antidote: Dimercaprol.

MERCUZANTHIN®, see Mercurophylline

MERETHOXYLLINE—Dicurin®
Mercurial diuretic. White amorphous solid. Commercial preparation contains Procaine to alleviate pain of injection.
Actions and Uses: As other mercurial diuretics, which see.
Warnings: See mercurial diuretics.
Administration: Intramuscular.
Preparations: Solution, 10%. Ampules, 1, 2 and 10 cc.
Antidote: Dimercaprol.

MERPHENYL NITRATE®, see
Phenylmercuric Nitrate

MERSALYL AND THEOPHYL-
LINE—Mersalyn®, Salyrgan-theophylline®

Mercurial diuretic. White powder, soluble in water.
Actions and Uses: Much same as all mercurial diuretics. Used mainly in treatment of congestive heart failure, reducing edema by increasing urinary output.
Warnings: Excessive use may lead to low-sodium syndrome. Contraindicated in acute nephritis. Intramuscular injections should be deep into the gluteal muscle. Paravenous infiltration may cause local necrosis.
Administration: Intramuscular, intravenous.
Preparations: Ampule, 10% solution with theophylline 5%, 1-2 cc.
Dose: 1-2 cc. as frequently as needed.
Antidote: Dimercaprol.

MERSALYN®, see Mersalyl and Theophyllin

MERTESTATE®, see Testosterone

MERTHIOLATE®, see Thimerosal

MESANTOIN®, see Methylphenylethylhydantoin

MESOPIN®, see Homatropine

MESTILBOL—Monomestrol®
Synthetic estrogen.
Actions and Uses: Same as other estrogenic substances, which see.
Warnings: See Estrogens.
Administration: Oral.
Preparations: Tablet, 0.5, 1.0 and 2.5 mg.
Dose: 0.5 to 2.5 mg. daily depending on condition.

MESTINON®, see Pyridostigmin

METAMINE®, see Triethanolamine trinitrate

METANDREN®, see Methyltestosterone

METAPHEN®, see Nitromersol

METARAMINOL—Aramine®
Adrenergic. One of the sympathomimetic amines used largely locally in the nasal mucosa to shrink it. Due to its intense vasoconstrictive action it also elevates the blood pressure. This property has been suggested as useful in the treatment of shock. The latter use remains to be evaluated. When used topically, however, its hypertensive action is to be considered. Said not to cause palpitations.

METHACHOLINE—Mecholyl®
Cholinergic. White crystals or powder, soluble in water. Available as chloride and bromide salts.
Absorption: From G. I. tract.
Actions and Uses: Reproduces effects of stimulation of vagus nerves. Slows heart, lowers blood pressure, increases tone of bladder and intestine. Used in urinary retention, abdominal distention, cardiac arrhythmias. Miotic in resistant cases.
Warnings: Parenteral use may cause severe reactions, especially contraindicated in asthmatic patients. Reactions may also include weakness, dizziness, nausea, vomiting and cardiac distress. Keep syringe with atropine dose at hand whenever using this drug parenterally. Use test dose first (2.5 mg.).
Administration: Oral, parenteral, iontophoresis (occasionally).
Preparations: Tablet, 0.2 Gm. Ampule, 25 mg. undissolved powder. Solution, ophthalmic.
Dose: Oral, 0.1–0.6 Gm. Intravenous, 10–25 mg.
Antidote: Atropine, 0.5–2 mg.

METHADON, see Methadone

METHADONE — Adanon®, Dolophine®, Methadon
Addictive analgesic.
Actions and Uses: Morphine substitute. Potent analgesic, but with real addiction potential. Nonsedative. May be used for replacement in morphine withdrawal. Suppresses cough.
Warnings: Addiction hazard is high. Narcotic laws must be followed.
Administration: Oral, subcutaneous.
Preparations: Tablet, 2.5 and 5 mg. Ampule, sterile solution, 1 cc. contains 10 mg.
Dose: Oral, for analgesia 2.5–10 mg.; for cough 1–2.5 mg. Subcutaneous, 2.5–10 mg.
Antidote: Nalorphine.

METHALLENESTRIL—Vallestril®
Synthetic estrogen. Not related to stilbestrol. See Estrogens.

Preparations: Tablet, 3 mg.
Dose: Of the order of 3-6 mg. daily, for menopausal symptoms.

METHA-MERDIAZINE®, see Trisulfapyrimidines

METHAMPHETAMINE—
A m p h e d r o x y n®, Desoxyephedrine®, Desoxyn®, Desyphed®, Dexoval®, Doxyfed®, Efroxine®, Methedrine®, Norodin®, Semoxydrine®, Syndrox®
Adrenergic, central nervous system stimulant. White crystals.
Actions and Uses: Has much the same actions as amphetamine (Benzedrine®) Central stimulation, with circulatory stimulation. Used in narcolepsy, parkinsonism, alcoholism and depressed states. Said also to depress appetite and used in the treatment of obesity.
Warnings: Produces insomnia, excitement. May elevate blood pressure. May cause dependence if used for prolonged periods.
Administration: Oral, intravenous.
Preparations: Tablet, 2.5, 5 mg. Sterile solution.
Dose: Oral, 2.5 to 5 mg. three times daily. Intravenous, 10–15 mg.
Antidote: Barbiturate.

METHAMPYRONE®, see Dipyrone

METHANOL, see Methyl Alcohol

METHANTHELINE—Banthine®
Antispasmodic, anticholinergic. The hydrochloride, white powder, soluble in water. Intensely bitter.
Absorption: From G. I. tract.
Actions and Uses: Same as atropine except action on stomach and intestinal tract is said to be so much more potent than its other parasympatholytic actions, that it is more convenient to use than atropine.
Warnings: Excessive action causes dryness of mouth, visual difficulties, stops perspiration and may elevate temperature. May cause flushing. There is a real danger of glaucoma in sensitive patients.
Administration: Oral, parenteral.
*Preparations*s Tablet, 25 mg., 50 mg.

Ampule, 50 mg. to be dissolved in 10 cc. before using.
Dose: 50–100 mg.

METHAPHENILENE—Diatrine®
One of the large series of antihistamine drugs, which see.

METHAPYRILENE—
Dormin®, Histadyl®, Semikon®, Thenylene®
One of the large series of antihistamine drugs, which see. This one in particular exerts strong sedative actions in many persons and, because of this, is now being sold without prescription under such names as Dormin® and Nytol®.

METHARBITAL—Gemonil®
Anticonvulsant barbiturate. White powder, slightly soluble in water.
Actions and Uses: Shares the anticonvulsant properties of phenobarbital and used, therefore, in epilepsy. Said to be effective in the various epileptic manifestations, grand mal, petit mal, myoclonic and mixed seizures. Its chief advantage, therefore, lies in its effectiveness in situations in which phenobarbital is ineffective.
Warnings: Although toxic effects are not common, may cause dizziness, rash, irritability, drowsiness, and gastric distress.
Administration: Oral.
Preparations: Tablet, 0.1 Gm.
Dose: 0.1 Gm. three times daily or less.
Antidote: Picrotoxin.

METHEDRINE®, see Methamphetamine

METHENAMINE—Urotropin®
Urinary antiseptic. White crystals or powder, soluble in water. Burns on ignition.
Actions and Uses: Methenamine alone is entirely inert. In highly acid urine, however, it liberates formaldehyde which exerts antiseptic action. Urine must be acid if it is to be effectual.
Warnings: May be irritant to urinary tract mucosa. Accessory drugs and diet may have to be arranged to make urine acid. Urinary acidity should be tested chemically. If urine fails to turn acid with drugs, renal function should be tested and the drug discontinued.

Administration: Oral.
Preparations: Tablet, 0.3 and 0.5 Gm.
There are also tablets which contain acidifying salts, but the more rational course is to use acidifying medication (such as ammonium chloride) separately.
Dose: 4–5 Gm. daily.
Antidote: If excessive reaction, use alkali such as sodium bicarbonate.

METHENAMINE MANDELATE— Mandelamine®
Urinary antiseptic.
A chemical combination of mandelic acid and methenamine with the theoretic advantages of combined action. See Methenamine and Mandelic Acid.

METHERGINE®, see Methylergonovine

METHIACIL®, see Methylthiouracil

METHIODAL—Skiodan®
Diagnostic. White powder, soluble in water.
Actions and Uses: Given intravenously, excreted by kidney and, since opaque to x-ray, used to visualize urinary tract. By rapidity of excretion also indicates kidney function to some extent. Also used in retrograde pyelography.
Warnings: Deteriorates in light. Contraindicated in severe renal and liver disease. Use carefully in patients with hyperthyroidism and tuberculosis. Contains iodine.
Administration: Intravenous, retrograde.
Preparations: Sterile solution, 20% and 40%.
Dose: Intravenous, 2 Gm. per 7 Kg. of body weight. Retrograde, 10–20 Gm. in 100 cc.

METHIONINE—Meonine®
Nutritional and lipotropic. Essential amino-acid present in casein and other protein-containing products. Also made synthetically.
Actions and Uses: Provides a specific factor to reverse fatty infiltration of liver. Used as dietary supplement and source of methionine in protein deficient patients, especially those exposed to indus-

trial or medicinal toxic agents, cirrhosis, treatment of hepatitis.
Administration: Oral, intravenous.
Preparations: Tablet, 0.5 Gm. Capsule, 0.5 Gm. Crystals, 50 Gm.
Dose: Oral, 3–20 Gm. daily. Intravenous, 5–10 Gm. by slow drip of 3% solution.

METHIUM®, see Hexamethonium

METHOCARBAMOL—Robaxin®
Skeletal muscle relaxant. Like all new drugs, especially of this type, long clinical trial is essential to establish its usefulness. Available in 0.5 Gm. tablets.

METHORPHINAN, see Racemorphan

METHOTREXATE®, see Amino-Methyl-Pteroylglutamic Acid

METHOXAMINE—Vasoxyl®
Adrenergic. Another of this long series of drugs. In this case the drug is said to exert a pressor action on blood pressure without cardiac acceleration.
Warnings: Although said not to have a direct action on the heart nor cerebral stimulating action, such a possibility is not entirely excluded. Elevation of blood pressure and bradycardia are, however, much more likely in excessive dosage. Use with especial care in patients with hypertension. See Epinephrine.

METHOXSALEN—Oxsoralen®, Xanthotoxin
New drug recommended for increasing pigmentation of the skin in vitiligo. Toxic potential may be high and drugs should be used with extreme caution. Dosage in the range of 20 mg. daily.

METHOXYPHENAMINE — Orthoxine®
One of the large series of adrenergic drugs, which see. Used especially for antiallergic action.

METHSCOPOLAMINE—Lescopine®, Pamine®, Skopolate®
Anticholinergic.
An atropine-like drug recommended for its action to relax G.I. spasm and to relieve G.I. hypermotility. Its actions and potential dangers are common to the

group. Dosage of the order of 15 mg. orally; 1.0 mg. parenterally. See Atropine.·

METHURITAL—Neraval®
Anesthetic. Ultra-rapid barbiturate, which see. Available in 1 and 2 Gm. vials for intravenous use.

METHYL ALCOHOL—Methanol, Wood Alcohol
Solvent. Clear colorless fluid with characteristic odor.
Actions and Uses: Highly toxic material used only as a solvent and never as medicament. Occasionally used as a substitute for ethyl alcohol with disastrous results, frequently blindness, acidosis and sometimes death.

METHYLAMINO-HYDROXY-METHYLHEPTANE—Aranthol®
New drug; sympathomimetic amine. Usefulness as such to be established but suggestion that it is a myocardial stimulant, seriously to be questioned.

METHYLBENZETHONIUM—Diaparene®
Antiseptic. Colorless crystals, bitter taste, soluble in water, the chloride.
Actions and Uses: A detergent antiseptic with limited trial as general antiseptic, used mainly in prevention of dermatitis in infants due to bacterial growth, especially ammonia splinters, in diapers.
Warnings: Take precautions to prevent accidental ingestion by infants. Remove wet diapers from infants. Soap inhibits disinfection by this agent. Therefore, thorough rinsing should precede its use.
Preparations: Tablet, 0.09 Gm.
Application: Dissolve one tablet in about 2 quarts of water. Pour over cleansed diapers and permit to dry.

METHYLCELLULOSE—Cellothyl®, Syncelose®
Laxative. White powder, swells in the presence of water.
Actions and Uses: Used to stimulate bowel activity, and hence, as a mild laxative by increasing intestinal bulk, and in attempting to relieve chronic constipation. Also presently used in edible non-caloric food-like wafers for weight reduction. Not especially effective.
Warnings: In common with all materials which increase intestinal bulk, should not be used when there is intestinal obstruction.
Administration: Oral.
Preparations: Powder. Combination with other drugs.
Dose: 1.5 Gm. three times daily.

METHYLENE BLUE
Urinary antiseptic and diagnostic. Blue powder, soluble in water.
Actions and Uses: A mild urinary antiseptic. Also used as a diagnostic dye. Formerly used in treatment of poisoning by cyanide and carbon monoxide.
Warnings: May cause nausea, vomiting, bladder irritation. Patients should be warned that urine will become green or blue.
Administration: Oral, intravenous.
Preparations: Tablet, 65, 130, 300 mg. Sterile solution, 2%.
Dose: Oral, 65–300 mg. Intravenous, 1.0 mg. per Kg. body weight.

METHYLERGONOVINE—Methergine®
Oxytocic. Partially synthesized derivative of ergonovine. Said to have effects which are somewhat more intense but of shorter duration than ergonovine, but otherwise much the same. See Ergonovine.

METHYLHEXANEAMINE — Forthane®
One of the large series of adrenergic drugs, which see. Used especially for antiallergic and nasal decongestant action.

METHYLPARAFYNOL—Dormison®
Hypnotic. Fluid in large greenish-blue capsule.
Actions and Uses: Claimed, without substantiation, to have actions as hypnotic superior to barbiturates.
Warnings: There is no reason to believe that danger of addiction is any less than in the case of barbiturates.
Administration: Oral.

Preparations: Soft gelatin capsule, 250 and 500 mg.
Dose: 250 to 500 mg.

METHYLPHENIDATE—Ritalin®

Stimulant. Central nervous stimulant said to increase alertness and improve mental outlook in depressed patients without affecting appetite or inducing insomnia. Action said to lie between that of Amphetamine and Caffeine. Position in therapy of this new drug remains to be determined. Available in 5 mg. (yellow.), 10 mg. (blue), 20 mg. (peach) tablets. Usual dose ranges around 10 mg. three times a day.

METHYL-PHENYLETHYL-HYDANTOIN—Mesantoin®

Anticonvulsant. White crystals, insoluble in water.
Actions and Uses: Much the same as diphenylhydantoin.

METHYL-PIPERIDYL-DIPHENYLGLYCOLATE—Cantil®

Anticholinergic. New drug; final position remains to be established. Available in 25 mg. tablets.

METHYLPREDNISOLONE—Medrol®

Anti-inflammatory hormone. New steroid closely related to prednisolone, which it also resembles pharmacologically. Available in 4 mg. tablets.

METHYLROSANILINE—
Pykotanin®, Gentian Violet, Crystal Violet

Antiseptic dye. Dark green powder, soluble in water, making a violet solution.
Actions and Uses: Used for antiseptic action in superficial infections, monilia infections, Vincent's infection, impetigo, furunculosis, dermatomycoses, pruritus, leukorrhea. Also used in pin worm, round worm and some fluke infestations.
Warnings: Stains skin and linen; may be removed with bleach. Patients should be instructed about staining and color. Contraindicated internally in patients with serious heart, liver or kidney dis-

eases. Nausea and even vomiting may occur after internal use.
Administration: Topical, oral.
Preparations: Tablet, 10 and 30 mg. Solution, 1%. Suppository 0.13 Gm.
Dose: Oral, 65 mg. three times daily. Topical, 1:500 to 1:1000.

METHYL SALICYLATE—
Wintergreen Oil

Flavor and analgesic. Colorless to reddish oily fluid, with characteristic odor and taste. Slightly soluble in water. There is no truth in the statement that there is any superiority of the natural material, derived from plants, over the synthetic material.
Absorption: Absorbed from skin.
Actions and Uses: Produces analgesia similar to other salicylates taken internally. Also used as a counterirritant.
Warnings: Excessive use may produce systemic toxicity. Especially serious poisoning occurs when ingested accidentally by children.
Administration: Topical.
Preparations: Ointment and solution.
Dose: Concentration, 10%.

METHYLTESTOSTERONE—Metandren®

Androgen. White crystals, insoluble in water.
Actions and Uses: Replaces, supplements natural male hormone in cases of testicular insufficiency, male menopause; in the female to suppress excessive menstrual bleeding, excessive swelling of breasts and other forms of excessive estrogenic activity. Used in treatment of undescended testicles. Especially useful because of oral and buccal absorption obviating injection.
Warnings: In male, should not be used for undescended testes under the age of 10–12 years. In the female, excessive dosage may induce virilism (masculinity). Contraindicated in treatment of male sterility and prostatic carcinoma. May induce relative sterility in the male, and in elderly patients, it may produce symptoms of heart failure.
Administration: Oral, sublingual.

Preparations: Capsule, 10–25 mg. Tablet, 5–10 mg.
Dose: Oral, 10–50 mg. depending on condition. Sublingual, 5 mg.

METHYLTHIOURACIL—Methiacil®, Muracil®, Thimecil®
Antithyroid. White crystals, slightly soluble in water.
Actions and Uses: Much the same as propylthiouracil, which see.

METHYPRYLON—Noludar®
Hypnotic. Another of the new central-depressant agents which has been introduced with major stress laid on the fact that it is not a barbiturate. Whether this drug has any real advantage as a hypnotic or sedative over barbiturates remains to be seen, but there is no reason to believe that the dangers of habitation are less.
Preparations: Tablet, 50 and 500 mg. Elixir, 50 mg. per teaspoonful.
Dose: Of the order of 100 mg.

METICORTELONE®, see Prednisolone

METICORTEN®, see Prednisone

METIMAZOLE—Tapazole®
Thiouracil derivative. Said to be about 15 times as potent as propylthiouracil; dosage ranges accordingly; dangers the same. Available in 5 and 10 mg tablets. See Thiouracil derivatives.

METOPON
Addictive analgesic.
Actions and Uses: Derivative of morphine which seems to have few, if any, advantages over morphine.
Warnings: See Morphine.
Administration: Oral.
Preparations: Capsule, 3 mg.
Dose: 3 mg.
Antidote: Nalorphine.

METRAZOL®, see Pentylenetetrazol

METUBINE®, see Dimethyl-tubocurarine

METYCAINE®, see Piperocaine

MICTINE®, see Aminometradine

MILIBIS®, see Glycobiarsol

MILK OF MAGNESIA, see Magnesia Magma

MILK SUGAR, see Lactose

MILONTIN®, see Phensuximide

MILTOWN®, see Meprobamate

MINERAL OIL, see Petrolatum

MIOKON®, see Diprotrizoate Sodium

MIOTICS
Physostigmine, Pilocarpine.

MIXED TOCOPHEROLS, see Vitamin E

MODERIL®, see Rescinnamine

MOEBIQUIN®, see Diiodohydroxyquinoline

MOL-IRON®, see Molybdenized Ferrous Sulfate

MOLOFAC®, see Dioctyl Sodium Sulfosuccinate

MOLYBDENIZED FERROUS SULFATE—Mol-Iron®
An iron complex claimed to have advantages over ferrous sulfate itself. These claims can only be established by long clinical experience; this is still wanting. Available in tablets containing 200 mg. ferrous sulfate and 3 mg. molybdenum oxide.

MONOBENZONE—Benoquin®
Pigment inhibitor. New drug suggested for treatment of hyperpigmentation due to melanin. Further experience is necessary for evaluation of utility as well as of dangers.

MONOBROMATED CAMPHOR
Convulsant.
Actions and Uses: Much the same as camphor.

MONOCAINE®, see Butethamine

MONODRAL®, see Penthienate

MONOMESTROL®, see Mestilbol

MORPHINE
Addictive analgesic. White fluffy powder, intensely bitter. The alkaloid is insoluble in water. The salts, sulfate and hydrochloride, are very soluble.
Actions and Uses: One of the most useful yet dangerous drugs. It is the best pain-

relieving agent available. Its action in this respect is a combination of a depression of pain appreciation and a euphoria (sense of well being) which reduces the patient's concern over his discomfort. It is the latter which gives morphine its special position, for often pain is impossible of complete relief without producing narcosis, but with this action of morphine, the patient is relieved of concern before such serious depths have been achieved. Drugs which are introduced as morphine substitutes either fail because they do not have this morphine action, or if they have it, they fail as substitutes because they have just as great an addiction potential as morphine. Whenever administering repeated doses of morphine for the relief of pain, it is well to inquire not only whether the patient has pain, but also whether he minds it.

Morphine also has the following actions which are useful therapeutically: it suppresses the cough reflex and hence, is used in cough mixtures; it decreases intestinal activity, hence is useful in the control of diarrhea; it stimulates the vagus nerve and thereby slows the heart and used in instances of rapid cardiac rates.

Warnings: Overdosage may cause serious depression of respiration. Frequent use may easily lead to addiction, especially in former addicts, alcoholics, depressed patients and otherwise unstable patients. May induce allergic reactions in patients with allergies. In acute pain in which diagnosis is in doubt, it may be well to withhold drug until diagnosis is established. Keep in locked cabinet. Narcotic laws require accounting of this drug's use. Intravenous use may be dangerous.

Administration: Oral, parenteral.

Preparations: Tablet. Sterile solution, for injection. Also used in cruder forms in tincture of opium and paregoric which contain much smaller amounts of morphine, but whose actions depend entirely on the morphine content. Pantopon® is a mixture of materials which derives virtually all its actions from the morphine content.

Dose: 4–30 mg., depending on indications.

Antidote: Nalorphine, Levallorphan.

MUCIN, see Gastric Mucin

MURACIL®, see Methylthiouracil

MUSCLE RELAXANTS, SKELETAL

Internuncial depressant: Mephenesin, Meprobamate, Methicarbamol, Orphenadrine, Promoxolane.

Curariform: Chondodendron Tomentosum Extract, Dimethyl-tubocurarine, Gallamine, Succinylcholine, Tubocurarine.

Anticholinergic: Benztropin, Caramiphen, Cycrimine, Procyclidine, Trihexyphenidyl.

Miscellaneous: Chlorpromazine, Diethazine, Diphenhydramine, Ethopropazine, Meprobamate, Promazine.

MUSTARD

Emetic and rubefacient. Brown powder, from mustard seed.

Actions and Uses: As a rubefacient, is used in the mustard plaster, which can be obtained in already prepared form or can be made from English mustard. Action is due to the oil in the powder. Also used as an emetic.

Warnings: Overdose may cause local and internal irritation.

Administration: Oral (emetic), external (plaster).

Preparations: Powder and prepared plaster.

Dose: Emetic, 15 Gm. shaken in a tumbler of water. Plaster, 2.5 Gm.

MUSTARGEN®, see Mechlorethamine

MYANESIN, see Mephenesin

MY-B-DEN®, see Adenosinemonophosphate

MYCIFRADIN®, see Neomycin

MYCOSTATIN®, see Nystatin

MYDRIATICS
Atropine, Belladonna, Eucatropine Homatropine, Phenylephrine.

MYLERAN®, see Busulfan

MYOCHRYSINE®, see Gold Sodium Thiomalate
MYOTEN®, see Mephenesin
MYOXANE®, see Mephenesin
MYRCIA OIL—Bay Oil
Flavor.
MYRISTICA OIL—Nutmeg Oil
Flavor and carminative. Pale yellow liquid, insoluble in water. Obtained from nutmeg.
Actions and Uses: Aromatic oil and carminative.
Warnings: May be highly irritant if undiluted.
Administration: Oral.
Preparations: Oil.
Dose: 0.03 cc.
MYRRH—Gum Myrrh
Protective and carminative. Yellowish to brownish fragments of resin.
Actions and Uses: Protective and stimulant to mucous membranes. Internally as a carminative.
Warnings: Overdosage may be irritant.
Administration: Topical, oral.
Preparations: Tincture.
Dose: Tincture, 2 cc.
MYSOLINE®, see Primidone
MYTELASE®, see Ambenonium

N

NAEPAINE—Amylsine®
Local anesthetic. Another of these drugs used principally as a local anesthetic in opthalmology when mydriasis is not desired.
NALLINE®, see Nalorphine
NALORPHINE—Nalline®
Antidote. The hydrochloride, white, soluble, odorless powder. Narcotic.
Actions and Uses: A derivative of morphine, therefore under Federal Narcotic Law. Pharmacologic antagonist to morphine, meperidine and methadone. Reverses respiratory depression, fall in blood pressure, cardiac arrhythmias, depression of reflexes and sleep pattern produced by overdosage with these de-

pressants. It is the best antidote for poisoning by them. It is ineffectual against depression produced by barbiturates and general anesthetics. It is not useful for the treatment of narcotic addiction.
Warnings: Until more is known about long-term effects should be used only for acute poisoning by the drugs indicated. Its use does not preclude the need for supportive therapy in serious depressions. In morphine addicts its use may be followed by typical withdrawal symptoms.
Administration: Intravenous, intramuscular, subcutaneous.
Preparations: Ampule containing 1 and 2 cc., 5 mg. per cc.
Dose: 5 to 10 mg. repeated in 10 to 15 minutes if necessary. May be repeated in 3 to 4 hours if necessary.
Antidote: In the case of serious withdrawal symptoms, the drug to which the patient is addicted.
NAPHAZOLINE—Privine®
Nasal decongestant. White powder with bitter taste. Hydrochloride, soluble in water.
Actions and Uses: Local vasoconstrictor with little action on the blood pressure. Causes reduction of swelling in nasal mucous membranes and used, therefore, in rhinitis, hay fever, etc. Action is somewhat more prolonged than most other nasal decongestants.
Warnings: Excessive use may lead to drowsiness, local mucous membrane irritation and "rebound" congestion.
Administration: Topical.
Preparations: Solution.
Dose: Concentration, 1:2000 dilution most frequently used, although 1:1000 solution is also available.
NAPHURIDE®, see Suramin
NAPRYLATE®, see Caprylic Compound
NARCOTICS Under Federal Control
Alphaprodine, Cannabis, Cocaine, Codeine, Dihydrocodeinone, Dihydromorphinone, Ethylmorphine, Heroin, Levorphan, Meperidine, Methadone, Metopon, Morphine, Opium, Pantopon®.

NARONE®, see Dipyrone

NARTATE®, see Dipyrone

NATRINIL®, see Carboxylic Resins

NEMBUTAL®, see Pentobarbital

NEO-ANTERGEN®, see Pyrilamine

NEOATOPHEN®, see Neocinchophen

NEOCALAMINE, PREPARED

Protective. Light orange powder (mainly zinc oxide, with 3% red ferric oxide and 4% yellow ferric oxide). Insoluble in water.

Actions and Uses: A skin protective and mild antiseptic used mainly in skin lotions and liniments. Generally preferred to calamine because of better color.

Warnings: Shake well, if in lotion. Store in well-stoppered containers.

Administration: Topical.

Preparations: Lotion and liniment.

Dose: Concentration, 1.5–3%.

NEOCINCHOPHEN—
Neoatophen®

Analgesic. White tasteless powder, insoluble in water.

Actions and Uses: Same action and uses as cinchophen, but is tasteless, largely because of its insolubility. Used mainly in gout.

Warnings: Dangers of liver damage and acute yellow atrophy the same as for cinchophen.

Administration: Oral.

Preparations: Tablet.

Dose: 0.3 Gm.

NEODROL®, see Stanolone

NEOHETRAMINE®, see Thonzylamine

NEO-HOMBREOL®, see Testosterone

NEOLIN®, see Benzathine Penicillin G

NEOHYDRIN®, see Chlormerodrin

NEO-IOPAX®, see Iodomethamate

NEOMYCIN—Mycifradin®

Antibiotic. White powder.

Absorption: Poorly absorbed from G. I. tract.

Actions and Uses: Antibacterial action against gram-positive and gram-negative organisms. Since it is poorly absorbed from G. I. tract, its action and usefulness is confined to the preparation of patients for G. I. tract surgery, where it is important to eliminate or suppress bacterial inhabitants of the bowel.

Warnings: Treatment before surgery should not extend over a period longer than 72 hours. Dispensed only on prescription.

Adminstration: Oral.

Preparations: Tablet, 0.5 Gm.

Dose: 1 Gm. given at intervals over a 24-48 hour period preoperatively.

NEONAL®, see Butethal

NEO-PENIL®, see Penethamate

NEO-SILVOL®, see Silver Iodide

NEOSTAM®, see Stibamine Glucoside

NEOSTIBOSAN®, see Ethylstibamine

NEOSTIGMINE—Prostigmin®

Cholinergic. White powder. The salts are soluble in water, usually the bromide and methyl sulfate.

Actions and Uses: Cause stimulation of parasympathetic nervous system by preventing the destruction of acetylcholine and thus causing it to accumulate in abnormal amounts in the body. Used to reduce muscle spasm in poliomyelitis, and in urinary retention and bowel ileus and megacolon. It also exerts an action which is useful in the treatment of myasthenia gravis and in relief of curarization.

Warnings: Excessive dosage may cause nausea, vomiting and depressed blood pressure. They induce asthmatic attack.

Administration: Oral, subcutaneous, intramuscular.

Preparations: Capsule, tablet, 1 mg. Ampule, 0.25 mg., 0.5 mg. Ophthalmic solution, 5%.

Dose: Oral, 1 mg. for children, 1.5 mg. for adults. Parenteral, 0.25 to 1.0 mg. subcutaneous or intramuscular.

Antidote: Atropine 2 mg. intravenously.

NEO-SYNEPHRINE®, see Phenylephrine

NEOTHYLLINE®, see Hyphylline

NERAVAL®, see Methurital

NERVOUS SYSTEM DEPRESSANTS
Anesthetics (general), Azacyclonal, Barbiturates, Chloral hydrate, Chlorpromazine, Ethchlorovynol, Ethinamate, Glutethimide, Hypnotics, Meprobamate, Methylparafynol, Methyprylon, Narcotics, Promazine, Rauwolfia derivatives, Sedatives, Tranquilizers.
Adrenergic drugs, Analeptics, Meratran, Methyl-Phenidylacetate.

NERVOUS SYSTEM STIMULANTS
Adrenergic drugs, Analeptics, Iproniazid, Methylphenidate, Pipradol.

NESACAINE®, see Chloroprocaine

NIACIN, see Nicotinic Acid

NIACINAMIDE, see Nicotinamide

NIADRIN®, see Isoniazid

NICONYL®, see Isoniazid

NICOTINAMIDE—Niacinamide
Vitamin. White powder with bitter taste. Soluble in water.
Absorption: Well absorbed from G. I. tract.
Actions and Uses: Same as nicotinic acid but does not produce the disagreeable peripheral flush, and for that reason is generally preferred in treatment of pellagra and vitamin B complex deficiencies.
Warnings: While overdosage is rarely possible, it is well to remember that rarely are vitamin deficiencies purely that of a single material and, therefore, that other vitamins are probably needed in the treatment of any vitamin deficiency.
Administration: Oral, parenteral.
Preparations: Tablet, 50 mg. Sterile solution, 50 mg. per cc., 100 mg. per cc.
Dose: Oral, 50-500 mg. in divided doses. Parenteral, 100 mg.

NICOTINIC ACID—Niacin
Vitamin. White powder, slightly soluble in water.

Absorption: Well absorbed from G. I. tract.
Actions and Uses: The specific antipellagra factor of the vitamin B complex, which also causes considerable peripheral flushing which many patients find disagreeable, though never a serious matter. Because of this, as a vitamin, it has been largely supplanted by nicotinamide, which has the same antipellagra value but does not produce the flush. On the other hand, the flushing action is used therapeutically in the attempt to improve peripheral circulation, and with reported success, in cases of acne vulgaris, Menière's syndrome, migraine headaches and multiple sclerosis.
Administration: Oral, parenteral.
Preparations: Capsule, tablet, 25 mg. Ampule, sterile solution 1 cc. containing 50 mg. and 100 mg.
Dose: Oral, 100 mg. Parenteral, 100 mg.

NICOZIDE®, see Isoniazid

NIKETHAMIDE—Coramine®
Analeptic. Colorless to pale yellow liquid. Miscible with water.
Actions and Uses: A convulsant drug, said to produce nervous system stimulation and by direct action on chemoreceptor reflex centers, stimulation of respiration and elevation of blood pressure. Used as respiratory and cardiac stimulant, for which action, however, there is little substantial proof, and in many circles, the drug has been largely discarded for more reliable ones.
Warnings: Overdosage may induce serious convulsions. Not to be used to the exclusion of oxygen and more acceptable stimulants in cases of respiratory and circulatory collapse.
Administration: Oral, parenteral.
Preparations: Tablet. Solution, ampules of sterile solution.
Dose: Oral, 0.5 Gm. Parenteral, 0.5 Gm.

NILEVAR®, see Norethandrolone

NISENTIL®, see Alphaprodine

NISULFAZOLE®, see Para-nitro-sulfathiazole

NITRANITOL®, see Mannitol Hexanitrate

NITRETAMIN®, see Triethanolamine Trinitrate

NITRIC ACID, FUMING—
Aqua Fortis, Fuming Nitric Acid
Acid. A highly caustic fuming liquid.
Actions and Uses: Used for its caustic action in the immediate treatment of animal bites for the prevention of rabies, and even this use is now in question.
Warnings: Internally, it is usually fatal. Contact with skin causes yellow discoloration which persists until the skin desquamates. Large amounts on skin will cause local necrosis. Keep in tightly stoppered bottle away from light. May turn yellow, but is still effective if it fumes.
Administration: Topical.
Preparations: The pure acid as described above.
Dose: In small amounts depending on size and depth of bite or wound.
Antidote: Alkali, sodium bicarbonate, used freely.

NITRITES
The nitrites as a group are used almost exclusively for relaxation of smooth muscle in spasm of coronary arteries in paroxysms of pain of angina pectoris. The action on blood vessels, however, is not limited to the coronary arteries alone, but is diffuse throughout the body and, as a consequence, use of these drugs may lead to a sharp fall in blood pressure. This may produce severe headaches, weakness, collapse, convulsions. It is fortunate, however, that severe reactions rarely develop in patients who require the action of these drugs, but far more commonly in patients who have no need for them. The development of headache is indication that the dose is too large for the patient.
Continued and too frequent use may lead to tolerance to the drug, but a few days abstinence is usually sufficient to bring about a return of the original susceptibility to the drug action. The difference between the various members of this group

is more in the speed of onset of action and duration than in the nature of the effect. The most commonly used members are nitroglycerin and amyl nitrite, largely because the effects develop so promptly, and because the pain of angina pectoris attacks are rarely of long duration.
Nitrites and organic nitrates: Amyl nitrite, Erythrityl tetranitrate, Inositol hexanitrate, Mannitol hexanitrate, Nitroglycerin, Pentaerythritol tetranitrate, Sodium nitrite, Triethanolamine trinitrate.

NITROFURANTOIN—Furadantin®
Urinary antiseptic. Yellow, bitter powder slightly soluble in alcohol and insoluble in water.
Absorption: Well absorbed from G.I. tract.
Actions and Uses: Wide spectrum of antibacterial activity, but does not inhibit fungi or viruses. Used as urinary antiseptic. See antiseptics.
Administration: Oral.
Warnings: Although said to have low index of toxicity, may induce nausea and vomiting. Contraindicated in cases with anuria, oliguria or severe kidney damage.
Preparations: Tablets, 50 and 100 mg.
Dose: 1 to 2 mg. per kilogram four times daily.

NITROFURAZONE—Furacin®
Antiseptic. Yellow crystalline powder, slightly soluble in water.
Actions and Uses: Possesses antibacterial activity in very dilute (1:200,000) form and is used topically in prophylaxis and treatment of superficial infections.
Warnings: Color changes with exposure to light but does not reduce effectiveness of drug. Continued use may lead to local reactions.
Administration: Topical.
Preparations: Ointment and solution.
Dose: Concentration, 0.2% or less.

NITROGEN MUSTARD, see Mechlorethamine

NITROGLYCERIN, see Glyceryl Trinitrate

NITROGLYN®, see Glyceryl Trinitrate

NITROLANS®, see Pentaerythritol Tetranitrate

NITROMERSOL—Metaphen®
Organic mercurial antiseptic. Yellow powder; dissolves in alkaline solutions. *Actions and Uses*: Far less irritant and corrosive than the inorganic mercurials. Used as a local antiseptic, especially as a household antiseptic.
Warnings: Not to be taken internally.
Administration: Topical.
Preparations: Tincture, solution, ophthalmic ointment, vaginal tampon.
Dose: Concentrations of 1:1000, 1:5000, 1:10,000.
Antidote: Dimercaprol.

NITROUS OXIDE—
Laughing Gas
Anesthetic. Colorless gas with a pleasant odor.
Actions and Uses: Produces analgesia and anesthesia by direct depression of central nervous system. Used for minor surgical procedures not requiring deep anesthesia, and for induction of surgical anesthesia, because it is more pleasant than the ether, which usually follows.
Warnings: This gas is used with little oxygen, the hypoxia during anesthesia may induce serious irreversible effects on the brain. Should not be used for patients with anemia, in shock, or serious circulatory defects.
Administration: Inhalation.
Preparations: Gas.
Dose: Concentration, 95%.

NOLUDAR®, see Methyprylon

NOR-EPINEPHRINE, see Levarterenol

NORETHANDROLONE—Nilevar®
Hormone. New corticosteroid said to reverse negative nitrogen balance, hence a restorative for weakness and emaciation due to illness and surgery. Usual effects of cortico-steroids not described for this drug. Usefulness in fatigue and weakness of unknown origin not established. Available in 10 mg. tablets. Dosage of the order of 30 to 50 mg. three times a day.

NORETHINDRONE—Norlutin®
Progestational hormone. New drug; value to be established. Available in 5 mg. tablets.

NORISODRINE®, see Isoproterenol
NORLUTIN®, see Norethindrone
NORODIN®, see Methamphetamine
NOSTYN®, see Ectylurea
NOVALDIN®, see Dipyrone
NOTEC®, see Chloral Hydrate
NOVATRIN®, see Homatropine
NOVOBIOCIN—Albamycin®,
Cathomycin®
Antibiotic. Obtained biosynthetically from cultures of *Streptomyces spheroides.*
Actions and Uses: Said to be highly effective against staphylococci and other bacteria resistant to penicillin.
Warnings: A new antibiotic whose indications, limitations and dangers are yet to be clearly delineated.
Administration: Oral.
Preparations: 250 mg. capsules.
Dose: 1.0 Gm followed by 250 mg. every 6 hours.

NOVOCAIN®, see Procaine
NPH INSULIN—Isophane Insulin
A mixture of rapidly and slowly acting forms of insulin, which see.
NUPERCAINE®, see Dibucaine
NUTMEG OIL, see Myristica Oil
NYDRAZID®, see Isoniazid
NYLIDRIN—Arlidin®
Vasodilator.
Actions and Uses: Recommended for intermittent claudication and vasospastic conditions to relieve pain and enhance peripheral circulation.
Warnings: A new drug; neither therapeutic value nor toxic potential fully established.
Administration: Oral, subcutaneous, intramuscular.
Preparations: Tablet, 6 mg. Ampule, 5 mg.
Dose: Oral, 18-24 mg. daily. Subcutaneous and intramuscular, 2.5-5 mg., 1-3 times daily.

NYSTATIN—Mycostatin®
Antibiotic. New antibiotic material said to be the first effective antifungal antibiotic. Effective against ano-rectal moniliasis which is reported as a complication of the use of the tetracycline antibiotics. Claimed to exert little toxicity. Further trial is needed to establish all its uses. Dosage of the order of 500,000 to 1,500,000 units daily.

NYTOL®, see Methapyrilene

O

OBSTETRICAL PITUITARY SOLUTION, see Pituitary, Posterior

OCTIN®, see Isometheptene

OIL, MINERAL, see Petrolatum

OIL OF CADE, see Juniper Tar

OIL OF MAIZE, see Corn Oil

OIL OF WINTERGREEN, see Methyl Salicylate

OILS, see also under name of oil.

OLEANDOMYCIN—Matromycin®
Antibiotic. New agent elaborated by *Streptomyces antibioticus.* Said to be effective against many organisms and strains of organisms resistant to the tetracyclines, particularly staphylococci, streptococci and pneumococci. In addition, it is said to have a very broad spectrum of activity on its own, including activity against some gram-negative bacteria, rickettsiae, large viruses and protozoa (notably amebae). How effective the drug is along these lines, and how long this effectiveness persists, remains to be established, although recent opinion is that it is definitely inferior to erythromycin against the staphylococcus. Available in 250 mg. capsules. Dosage of the order of 1 to 2 capsules 3 to 4 times a day. The dangers of continued treatment are probably the same as for other Antibiotics, which see.

OLEIC ACID
Base.
Actions and Uses: A liquid acid used as a basis for ointments.

OLEORESIN OF ASPIDIUM, see Aspidium Oleoresin

OLEORESIN OF MALE FERN, see Aspidium Oleoresin

OLEOVITAMIN A
Vitamin A. A thin oily liquid.
Actions and Uses: Supplies vitamin A. Deficiency results in skin, mucous membrane changes, changes in the eyes, xerophthalmia, keratosis, and reduction in dark vision.
Warnings: Overdosage may cause loss of weight, irritability, rash, loss of hair and tenderness.
Administration: Oral.
Preparations: Capsule, tablet. Solution. Concentrate. Mixtures with other vitamins.
Dose: Adult, 25,000 Units daily.

OLEOVITAMIN D, SYNTHETIC, see Synthetic Oleovitamin D

OLIVE OIL
Nutritional. Pale yellow oil with characteristic taste and odor.
Actions and Uses: A common food which, despite its reputation, has no special virtues other than its characteristic taste, over a large number of common and less expensive oils. Has no special medical properties.
Warnings: Overdosage may cause nausea and diarrhea.

OPIUM
Addictive analgesic. Flattened masses with bitter taste and characteristic odor.
Actions and Uses: Opium, although containing a mixture of alkaloids, derives its essential actions from its morphine content, which comprises about 10% of its weight. It has no particular actions which cannot be derived from the pure morphine. Preparations are most frequently used for cough and diarrhea.
Warnings: Has all the dangers of morphine.
Administration: Oral.

Preparations: Crude opium, extract, granulated opium, powdered opium, tincture of opium (10% opium, i.e., 1% morphine) and camphorated tincture of opium (paregoric, contains 4% tincture of opium, therefore, each cc. contains 0.4 mg. morphine).
Dose: Varies with indications.
Antidote: Nalorphine.

ORADIOL®, see Ethinyl Estradiol

ORAL FAT EMULSION—Ediol®
Nutritional. Finely divided particles of fat in an emulsion.
Actions and Uses: A source of fat which can be used to supplement the diet either in the diet or by stomach tube. Useful in malnutrition of various causes.
Warnings: Overdosage may lead to diarrhea. Small doses only may be acceptable in fat intolerance.
Administration: Oral, added to food or by stomach tube.
Preparations: Emulsion containing 50% fat (coconut oil) and 12.5% sucrose.
Dose: As indicated by weight of patient and condition.

ORANGE OIL—Sweet Orange Oil
Flavor. Yellow orange liquid.
Actions and Uses: Aromatic flavor characteristic of orange peel.
Administration: Oral.
Preparations: Compound spirit of orange.

ORANGE PEEL, BITTER
Flavoring agent.
Actions and Uses: Made from unripe and ripe peel of orange and used as flavoring agent.

ORANGE PEEL, SWEET,
  see Orange Peel, Bitter

ORANIXON®, see Mephenesin

ORESTRALYN®, see Ethinyl Estradiol

ORETON®, see Testosterone

ORINASE®, see Tolbutamide

ORPHENADRINE—Disipal®
Skeletal muscle relaxant. New drug; final position as a therapeutic agent to be established. Available in 50 mg. tablets.

ORRIS
Powder base.

Largely discarded because it is highly allergenic.

ORTAL®, see Hexethal

ORTHOXINE®, see Methoxyphenamine

OUABAIN—G-Strophanthin
Cardiac stimulant. Crystalline powder, slightly soluble in water.
Absorption: Poorly absorbed from G. I. tract.
Actions and Uses: Actions virtually identical with digitalis, with these differences: (1) not absorbed from intestinal tract and not given orally; (2) by parenteral injection it develops its effects more rapidly than any other digitalis material in common use. Used primarily when rapid effects are needed. See Digitalis.
Warnings: Same as all digitalis materials.
Administration: Intramuscular, intravenous.
Preparations: Solution, ampules containing 0.25, 0.5, 1.0 mg. per cc.
Dose: 0.25 to 1.0 mg. given as needed.

OVOCYLIN®, see Estradiol

OX BILE EXTRACT—Bile Salts
Digestive. Greenish or brownish powder with bitter taste. Contains dehydrocholic and taurocholic acids which as such are often used for the same reasons and with much the same results as the crude ox bile.
Actions and Uses: Stimulates evacuation of gall-bladder and substitutes for bile in digestion in diseases in which the bile is deficient.
Warnings: Do not chew tablets. May cause diarrhea.
Administration: Oral.
Preparations: Tablet, 65 mg.
Dose: 0.2 to 0.3 Gm., 3 times daily.

OXOPHENARSINE—Mapharsen®
Antiluetic. White powder, soluble in water.
Actions and Uses: Treatment of early syphilis. Now largely replaced by penicillin. As effective as penicillin but not as convenient.
Warnings: See Arsenic.
Administration: Intravenous.

Preparations: Ampule, 60 mg. to be dissolved before using.
Dose: 45 mg.
Antidote: Dimercaprol.

OXSORALEN®, see Methoxsalen

OXTRIPHYLLINE—Choline Theophyllinate, Choledyl®
Xanthine. Recommended, without good evidence, as superior to other theophylline drugs for the relief of anginal pain as well as in asthma. Final position yet to be established. Dosage ranges about the same as for Aminophylline.

OXUCIDE®, see Piperazine

OXYGEN
Essential gas. Colorless, odorless gas.
Actions and Uses: When administered in high concentrations, increases amount of oxygen dissolved in blood, and thus makes available more oxygen to tissues. Used in diseases such as pneumonia and physiologic conditions such as vascular collapse, in which there is insufficient oxygen made available to tissues. Used in carbon monoxide poisoning.
Warnings: Highly inflammable. Keep away from flames and sparks.
Administration: Inhalation, by catheter, mask or tent, the last being by far the most pleasant, although mask is efficient.
Preparations: Cylinders.
Dose: Pure oxygen should be given for relatively short period of time, but concentrations of 70% or less are well tolerated. Inhalation must be given over long periods of time (hours) to be of particular value.

OXYPHENONIUM—Antrenyl®
One of the long list of anticholinergic drugs with much the same actions and dangers as atropine, which see.

OXYPOLYGELATIN—Plazmoid®
Parenteral fluid. Beef-bone collagen converted into blood substitute with electrolyte.
Actions and Uses: A substitute for blood and plasma where these are not available or, for one reason or another cannot be used. Requires no typing.

Warnings: Has not yet had wide-scale trial. Inject slowly.
Administration: Intravenous.
Preparation: Infusion bottles, 500 or 1000 cc.
Dose: As required by situation.

OXYTETRACYCLINE — Terramycin®
Antibiotic. Greenish-yellow powder derived from *streptomyces rimosus.*
Actions and Uses: One of the so-called broad spectrum antibiotics, effective against a large variety of common disease producing bacteria and some viruses as well. Most important among the latter are those of virus (primary atypical) pneumonia. Also many rickettsial infections. Closely resembles aureomycin in all properties.
Warnings: Liquid preparations deteriorate. Store in refrigerator. Store dry preparations in dry, cool place. May cause G.I. upsets, skin and peri-anal and vulvar rashes. Gastric distress may sometimes be avoided by taking directly after meals.
Administration: Oral, intramuscular, intravenous.
Preparations: Capsule, 50, 250 mg. Drops, in vial to be dissolved before using. Elixir, 50 mg. per cc. Sterile solution, to be dissolved before using, 250 and 500 mg., with sodium glycinate; to make at least 100 cc.
Dose: Oral, 500 mg. every hours. Intravenous, 0.5 to 1.0 Gm. daily in divided doses.

OXYTOCICS
Ergot, Ergotamine, Ergonovine, Methyl ergonovine, Oxytocin, Posterior Pituitary.

OXYTOCIN—Pitocin®
Oxytocic. Sterile soluble containing the active oxytocic principle.
Absorption: Not absorbed from G. I. tract.
Actions and Uses: Stimulates uterine contraction. Used in obstetrics to induce labor and stop postpartum hemorrhage.
Warnings: May induce symptoms of shock in sensitive patients.
Administration: Intramuscular.

Preparations: Ampule, 10 oxytocic units per cc.
Dose: 0.2 to 1.0 cc. (2–10 U.S.P. units).
Antidote: Epinephrine, for shock.

P

P³², see Radiophosphate Sodium
PABA, see Para-aminobenzoic Acid
PACATAL®, see Mepazine
PAGITANE®, see Cycrimine
PALUDRINE®, see Chloroguanide
PAMAQUINE—Plasmochin, Plasmoquine
Antimalarial. In little use at present.

PAMINE®, see Methscopolamine
PAMISYL®, see Para-Aminosalicylic Acid

PANCREATIN
Digestive. Cream colored powder, incompletely soluble in water.
Actions and Uses: For predigestion of starchy and protein foods.
Warnings: Destroyed by gastric acidity. Give in enteric coated pills.
Administration: Oral.
Preparations: Tablet, enteric coated.
Dose: 0.5 Gm.

PANPARNIT®, see Carmiphen
PANMYCIN®, see Tetracycline, Phosphate Buffered
PANTOPAQUE®, see Iophendylate®

PANTOPON®
Addictive analgesic. Mixture of narcotic alkaloids naturally occuring in opium, about one-fifth morphine, but altered so as to be readily dissolved in water. All its important effects are derived from its morphine content and it has no real advantages over morphine other than its name which is not generally associated with morphine in the mind of the layman. This makes it often possible to prescribe a potent narcotic with the patient and relatives remaining in ignorance of its real nature.

Warnings: See Morphine.
Antidote: Nalorphine.

PAPAVERINE
Vasodilator. White crystals, soluble in water. Bitter taste. Usually the hydrochloride.
Absorption: From the G. I. tract.
Actions and Uses: Relaxes smooth muscle. Used in vasospastic conditions, such as spasm of blood vessels in coronary thrombosis, vascular occlusions, embolisms, etc. In the conditions for which it is used, the situation is often irreversible and therefore, little may be expected from the drug in such instances.
Warnings: Narcotic. Overdosage may cause faintness. Inject slowly. Do not use if solution is unclear.
Administration: Oral, intravenous.
Preparations: Tablet, 60 mg. Ampule, containing 1–2 cc., 30 mg. per cc.
Dose: 30–100 mg.

PARA-AMINOBENZOIC ACID— PABA
Antirickettsial. White or yellow powder, slightly soluble in water.
Absorption: Absorbed from G. I. tract.
Actions and Uses: Depresses activity of certain rickettsial infections and used in their treatment. Antagonizes the sulfonamides; should not be used together with them.
Warnings: Reduces effectiveness of sulfonamides.
Administration: Oral.
Preparations: Tablet.
Dose: 0.5 as dietary supplement; about 20 Gm. daily as antirickettsial agent.

PARA-AMINOSALICYLIC ACID— Pamisyl®, PAS, Pasem®, Para-Pas®, Parasal®, Propasa®
Antitubercular. White powder, sodium and potassium salts soluble in water.
Absorption: Absorbed from G. I. tract.
Actions and Uses: When used with streptomycin in treatment of tuberculosis, it enhances its potency and delays the development of bacilli resistant to the streptomycin.
Warnings: May produce toxic effect in liver and kidney. Sometimes causes loss

of appetite, nausea, vomiting. These latter symptoms are less common when the drug is taken together with food.
Administration: Oral.
Preparations: Solution, 20%. Tablet, 0.5 Gm. of the acid form.
Dose: 10–15 Gm. daily in four doses.

PARABROMDYLAMINE—
Dimetane®
Another of the large series of antihistaminics, which see. Relative importance remains to be established by clinical experience. Available in 4 mg. tablets, 12 mg. long-action tablets, and elixir.

PARACODIN®, see Dihydrocodeinone

PARACORT®, see Prednisone

PARACORTOL®, see Prednisolone

PARADIONE®, see Paramethadione

PARAFFIN
Base for ointments. White transluscent mass, insoluble in water. Softens and melts by gentle heat.
Actions and Uses: Used to raise melting point, i.e. to harden, ointments, to give stiffness to dressings and for covering skin grafts. Not used internally.

PARAFORMALDEHYDE—
Trioxymethylene
Fumigant.
Actions and Uses: A tablet which when heated, liberates free formaldehyde gas. Used for sterilization. Effective treatment requires about 12 hours.
Warnings: Gas is highly irritant. Avoid inhalation. Keep pastilles in tightly stoppered, dry container and store in cool place.

PARALDEHYDE
Sedative. Colorless liquid with characteristic and highly disagreeable taste and pungent penetrating odor. Soluble in water.
Actions and Uses: A potent sedative and hypnotic, producing its effects fairly promptly after oral administration. Its taste, and the fact that it is partly excreted through the lungs, giving the breath its characteristic odor for several hours, is one of the main reasons for its restricted use. Commonly used for noisy and obstreperous alcoholics because of its prompt and effective action.
Warnings: Use with caution in liver disease. Rapid injection may cause pulmonary edema or cardiac failure. Overdosage may cause profound coma, respiratory depression, toxic hepatitis.
Administration: Oral, rectal, intramuscular, intravenous.
Preparations: Undiluted liquid.
Dose: Oral, 2–6 cc. Rectal, 10–20 cc. diluted with bland oil. Intravenous, 2–5 cc. Intramuscular, 2–7.5 cc.
Antidote: Analeptics such as picrotoxin.

PARAMETHADIONE—Paradione®
Anticonvulsant. Clear colorless liquid, not miscible with water.
Actions and Uses: Much the same as trimethadione and hence, used mainly in treatment of petit mal.
Warnings: See Trimethadione.
Preparations: Capsule, 0.3 Gm. Solution, 0.3 Gm. per cc.
Dose: 0.9 Gm. in divded doses daily.

PARAMINYL®, see Pyrilamine

PARA-NITROSULFATHIAZOLE—
Nisulfazole®
A sulfonamide usually injected rectally for local action in the rectum. See Sulfonamides.

PARA-PAS®, see Para-Aminosalicylic Acid

PARASAL®, see Para-Aminosalicylic Acid

PARATHYROID
Hormone. A solution of the hormone standardized in U.S.P. Units; obtained from parathyroid glands of cattle.
Absorption: Not absorbed from G. I. tract.
Actions and Uses: Mobilizes calcium from bones. Used in treatment of convulsions due to lack of natural hormone (hypoparathyroidism) of whatever cause. Rarely, also, used in internal hemorrhage, in nephritic edema and for removal of lead in lead poisoning.
Warnings: Overaction may cause severe

G. I. disturbances, depression of central nervous system or damage to organs due to abnormal deposition of calcium. Dangerous in use for lead poisoning because it may precipitate lead colic or encephalopathy.
Administration: Subcutaneous, intravenous.
Preparations: Ampule, containing 100 units per cc.
Dose: 20–40 Units twice a day; more in emergencies.

PARAZINE®, see Piperazine

PAREDRINE®, see Hydroxyamphetamine

PAREGORIC, see Camphorated Tincture of Opium

PARENAMINE®, see Amino Acid Preparations

PARENTERAL FLUIDS
Electrolyte solutions: Ammonium chloride, Plasma Expanders, Potassic Saline, Potassium chloride, Saline (isotonic, hypertonic), Sodium lactate, Ringer's.
Blood derivatives: Antihemophilic plasma, Normal human plasma (dried), Normal human plasma (citrated), Normal human serum, Normal human serum albumin, Normal human serum albumin (salt poor).
Plasma expanders: Dextran, Oxypolygelatin, Polyvidone.

PARENTRACIN®, see Bacitracin

PARENZYME®, see Trypsin, Crystalline

PARSIDOL®, see Ethopropazine

PAS, see Para-Aminosalicylic Acid

PASEM®, see Para-Aminosalicylic Acid

PASKALIUM®, see Potassium Aminosalicylate

PASKATE®, see Potassium Aminosalicylate

PATHILON®, see Tridihexide

PAVERIL®, see Dioxyline

PEACH KERNEL OIL, see Persic Oil

PEANUT OIL—Arachis Oil
Nutritional and vehicle. Pale yellow oil with bland taste.
Actions and Uses: Solvent, base, food.
Warnings: Overdose may cause diarrhea. Same as other edible oils.
Administration: Oral, in external medications. Parenteral, solvent for oil-soluble parenteral medications.

PECTIN—Andira®
Emulsant. For emulsifying cod liver oil, and in treatment of diarrheas. Use as a medicament is decreasing, but use for pharmaceutic preparations is increasing.
Actions and Uses: For emulsifying cod liver oil, and in treatment of diarrheas. Use as a medicament is decreasing, but use for purpose of pharmaceutic preparation increasing.

PEGANONE®, see Ethotoin

PENETHAMATE—Neo-Penil®
Antibiotic. A new salt of penicillin G.
Actions and Uses: Said to produce higher concentrations in lung tissue than other forms of penicillin. Otherwise its actions and duration of action is much the same as procaine penicillin G. May be especially useful in pulmonary disease.
Administration: Intramuscular.
Warnings: Same as for other penicillin preparations.
Dose: 500,000 Units.

PENICILLIN
Antibiotic. White powder, soluble in water. Dose expressed in units. 1000 Units equal to 0.6 mg. of pure crystalline penicillin.
Absorption: About 20% of oral dose is absorbed from G. I. tract.
Actions and Uses: Most potent antibacterial material in medicine. Effective against wide variety of common pathogenic bacteria. Effective by many routes of administration. Fairly rapidly eliminated in urine. One of the most benign (nontoxic) drugs in medicine in relation to its effective dose. There are several varieties of penicillin of which penicillin G is the one of choice.
Warnings: Highly allergenic, especially

when applied topically. Causes severe urticaria in sensitive patients. Oral administration may cause diarrhea and loss of appetite. Injections of crystalline penicillin intramuscularly may be painful; intravenously, may cause thrombosis.

Administration: Oral, rectal (not recommended), intramuscular, intravenous (in urgent cases), topical, inhalation (in nebulae) and into body cavities (joint, cerebro-spinal, etc.).

Preparations: Although the preparations on the market are so numerous as to be completely befuddling, there are only a few fundamentally different varieties of penicillin.

There are a few preparations of the mixed amorphous penicillins but in most instances, to insure purity and constancy, preparations are derived from crystalline penicillin G, which may be had in the soluble and quickly absorbed potassium, sodium and calcium salts.

Repository forms are more commonly used. These provide adequate blood levels but require fewer injections than the crystalline form because of slow absorption after injection. Repository forms are available suspended in oil, beeswax (largely discarded), as procaine penicillin and as a mixture of crystalline and procaine penicillin.

Oral forms usually come in tablets containing buffering materials to counteract gastric acidity.

Prompt brief action: Calcium penicillin, Crystalline potassium penicillin G, Crystalline sodium penicillin G, Sodium penicillin.

Prolonged action: Aluminum penicillin, Benzathine, Crystalline procaine penicillin G (aqueous suspension, oily suspension), Ephenamine, Penicillin G, Hydrabamine penicillin G, Phenoxymethyl hydrabamine penicillin.

Oral: Tablet, together with buffering agent to counteract the destructive action of gastric acid on penicillin. Solution, for use in children. Troches, for local action in mouth and throat. Phenoxymethyl penicillin (Penicillin V) is an especially well and rapidly absorbed form of penicillin. Phenoxymethyl hydrabamine penicillin is a well absorbed oral form with prolonged action.

Rectal: Suppository, not recommended because of unreliable effects.

Inhalation: Powder, for use in nebulizers, crystalline or procaine.

Topical: Ointment, usually amorphous or crystalline penicillin.

Antiallergic: Benzathine and Ephenamine said to be less allergenic than unaltered penicillin or penicillin G.

Dose: Depending on condition and mode of administration. For an infection such as pneumonia of average severity, an intramuscular dose of 300,000 units a day of repository penicillin would be administered. In any situation in which penicillin is administered orally, the dose is generally 5 times as large as the intramuscular dose.

PENICILLIN G, see Penicillin

PENICILLIN O, see Potassium Penicillin O

PENICILLIN V, see Phenoxymethyl Penicillin

PENTAERYTHRITOL TETRANITRATE—Angicap®, Nitrolans®, Peritrate®

Vasodilator. White crystalline material, insoluble in water.

Actions and Uses: Same group as nitroglycerin in treatment of precordial pain of angina pectoris. Effective in reducing frequency of attacks and therefore, used in the prophylaxis of angina pectoris.

Warnings: Side effects may occur occasionally: headache, nausea, rash.

Administration: Oral.

Preparations: Tablet, 10 mg.

Dose: 10 mg. 3–4 times daily.

PENTAQUINE

Antimalarial. Yellow powder with bitter taste. Soluble in water. Usually the phosphate.

Absorption: Absorbed from G. I. tract.

Actions and Uses: Used only in cases of relapsing malaria. Too toxic for use as prophylaxis and in average case for therapy. Often used together with quinine. *Warnings*: Toxic effects: **abdominal cramps**, loss of appetite, methemoglobinemia, hypotension, nausea, vomiting. May damage kidneys. Contraindicated in severe renal disease. *Administration*: Oral. *Preparations*: Tablet and capsule. *Dose*: 30 mg. daily in divided doses.

PENTHIENATE—Monodral®
Anticholinergic. The bromide. Available in 5 mg. capsules. Dosage 1-2 capsules. See Anticholinergic drugs.

PENTOBARBITAL— Nembutal®
Hypnotic and barbiturate. White powder, soluble in water. Bitter taste.
Absorption: From G. I. tract.
Actions and Uses: Similar to those of the other barbiturates. Intermediate in rapidity with which it induces hypnosis and in length of duration of effects.
Warnings: May induce dependence if used regularly. Used frequently in suicidal attempts.
Administration: Oral, intravenous.
Preparations: Capsule, yellow, 100 mg. Ampule, 50 mg. in 5 cc.
Dose: Oral, 0.1 Gm. Intravenous, variable, up to 0.5 Gm.
Antidote: Analeptics such as picrotoxin.

PENTOLINIUM—Ansolysen®
A new ganglionic blocking agent with much the same type of effects as hexamethonium, which see, but said to be less toxic and to exert a more prolonged action. More experience is required to evaluate this new agent. Available in 40 and 100 mg. tablets, and ampules, 10 mg. per cc. Dosage must be carefully controlled by observations of blood pressure as well as toxic effects.

PENTOTHAL®, see Thiopental

PENTYLENETETRAZOL— Cardiazol®, Metrazol®
Analeptic. White crystals, bitter taste, soluble in water and alcohol.
Actions and Uses: Convulsant and stimulant of midbrain and spinal cord. Used as convulsant in schizophrenia and other psychologic derangements, to accelerate recovery in narcosis, especially in barbiturate poisoning.
Warnings: During violent convulsions accidents, especially fractures of vertebrae, may occur. Overdosage in narcotized patients may lead to serious poisoning by the antidote.
Administration: Intravenous.
Preparations: 1-3 cc. ampules containing 0.1 Gm. per cc.
Dose: 0.1-0.3 Gm.
Antidote: Barbiturates.

PEN-VEE®, see Phenoxymethyl Penicillin

PEPPERMINT
Flavor.
Actions and Uses: Carminative and flavor.
Warnings: Containers should be kept tightly stoppered.
Administration: Oral.
Preparations: Oil. Spirit, 1%. Water, a saturated solution of the oil.
Dose: Oil, 0.1 cc. Spirit, 0.1 cc. Water, 15 cc.

PEPSIN
Digestive. Yellowish powder, soluble in water.
Actions and Uses: To assist in digestion of proteins; an action of limited questionable utility.
Administration: Oral.
Preparations: Elixir, saccharated pepsin.
Dose: 0.5 Gm.

PERANDREN®, see Testosterone

PERAZIL®, see Chlorcyclizine

PERCORTEN®, see Desoxycorticosterone

PERICLOR®, see Petrichloral

PERIN®, see Piperazine

PERITRATE®, see Pentaerythritol Tetranitrate

PERMAPEN®, see Benzathine Penicillin G

PERNOSTON®, see Butallylonal

PEROXIDE, see Hydrogen Peroxide

PERPHENAZINE—Trilafon®
Tranquilizer. Chlorpromazine congener,

with much the same actions and dangers. Final position in therapeutic use will be established only after long clinical trial. Available in 2, 4, 8 and 16 mg. tablets.

PERSIC OIL—Apricot Kernel Oil, Peach Kernel Oil
Actions and Uses: Same as for expressed almond oil.

PERUVIAN BALSAM
Vehicle and skin stimulant. Dark brown viscid liquid.
Actions and Uses: Used in ointments. Mildly antiseptic and stimulant to healing of indolent ulcers.
Administration: Topical.
Preparations: Ointment.
Dose: Concentration, 10%.

PETRICHLORAL—Periclor®
Sedative. Similar to Chloral Hydrate, which see. Dosage much the same.

PETROLATUM
Base for ointments, vehicle and laxative. Colorless, tasteless, odorless, solid, semisolid or liquid.
Actions and Uses: Base or vehicle in ointments, sprays, etc. Laxative in constipation. Not absorbed and of no nutritive value.
Warnings: May prevent absorption of fat soluble vitamins in food. Inhalation may cause lipoid pneumonia.
Administration: Topical, oral.
Preparations: Jelly. White petrolatum. Liquid (light and heavy) usually called mineral oil. Differing only in melting point. Also available in emulsions and mixtures with agar-agar, etc.
Dose: Oral, 15-30 cc.

PETROLEUM BENZINE—
Petroleum Ether
Solvent. Clear inflammable liquid.
Actions and Uses: Grease solvent. Preparation of skin for surgery.
Warnings: Highly inflammable. Not to be used internally. Highly toxic, causing confusion, dizziness, blood dyscrasias, drowsiness, vomiting, fever, bronchitis.

PETROLEUM ETHER, see
Petroleum Benzine

PHANODORN®, see Cyclobarbital

PHARMACEUTICALS
These comprise a large number of materials without significant pharmacodynamic action but which are used in the physical preparation of medicaments. Most of these agents are not listed here.

PHEMEROL®, see Benzethonium

PHENACAINE—Holocaine®
Surface anesthetic. White crystals with bitter taste. Slightly soluble in water. Usually the hydrochloride.
Absorption: Absorbed from surface of mucous membranes.
Actions and Uses: Drops in eye quickly produce local anesthesia. Use as a local anesthetic is largely restricted to eye.
Warnings: Highly toxic by intravenous injection.
Administration: Topical.
Preparations: Solution.
Dose: Concentration, 1%.

PHENACEMIDE—Phenurone®
Anticonvulsant. White tasteless powder, slightly soluble in water.
Actions and Uses: Anticonvulsant, effective in all forms of epilepsy.
Warnings: A new drug with serious side effects, personality changes, hepatic damage, bone marrow depression. To be used only by those with experience with such drugs.
Administration: Oral.
Preparations: Tablet, 0.5 Gm.
Dose: 1 to 2 Gm. daily in divided doses.

PHENACETIN, see Acetophenetidin

PHENACRIDANE—Acrizane®
Antifungal. New agent, value yet to be established.

PHENAGLYCODOL—Ultran®
Tranquilizer. Originally studied as an anticonvulsant; value as such or as a tranquilizer remains to be established by long clinical trial. Available in 300 mg. tablets.

PHENARSONE—Aldarsone®
Antiprotozoal and arsenical. White powder, soluble in water, the sulfoxylate.
Actions and Uses: An arsenical with antiluetic and antiprotozoal activity. Used

in *Trichomonas vaginalis* infections and occasionally in syphilis of the central nervous system.
Warnings: See arsenic.
Administration: Intravenous, intravaginal.
Preparations: Ampule, 1 Gm., to be dissolved in 10 cc. sterile distilled water. Powder, 0.5 Gm. with kaolin for insufflation. Suppository, 0.13 Gm.
Dose: Depends on indication.
Antidote: Dimercaprol.

PHENAZONE, see Antipyrine

PHENAZOTHIADIAZOLE— Urosulfin®
Sulfonamide. Recommended principally as a urinary antiseptic. Advantages over other similar drugs remain to be established.

PHENERGAN®, see Promethazine

PHENETSAL—Salophen®
Non-addictive analgesic. No evidence of real superiority over any of the standard analgesics of this series that have been in use long. Available in 0.3 Gm. tablets.

PHENINDAMINE—Thephorin®
One of the large series of antihistamine drugs, which see.

PHENINDIONE—Danilone®, Hedulin®
Anticoagulant. Not a coumarin derivative.
Actions and Uses: A relatively new anticoagulant with much the same actions and uses as the coumarin anticoagulants, which see. Action develops and disappears more rapidly than that of dicumarol. May have special value in instances in which the coumarin derivatives must be avoided.
Warnings: See Bishydroxycoumarin.
Administration: Oral.
Preparations: Tablet, 25 mg.
Dose: Dosage must be followed and guided by daily observations on the prothrombin levels in the blood. Initially about 200 mg. in the first 24 hours, thereafter about 25 mg. twice daily.
Antidote: Vitamin K, 50–100 mg. intravenously.

PHENIRAMINE—Trimeton®
One of the large series of antihistamine drugs, which see.

PHENMETRAZINE—Preludin®
Adrenergic. Recommended as appetite depressant. The nature of this action is not clear but is probably the same as that of amphetamine. Value as appetite depressant remains to be established. Available in 25 mg. tablets.

PHENOBARBITAL—Luminal®
Hypnotic and barbiturate. White powder, bitter taste, slightly soluble in water. The sodium salt is very soluble.
Absorption: From G. I. tract.
Actions and Uses: Same as other barbiturates. As compared with most, action develops slowly and persists for a relatively long period of time. Especially effective in preventing convulsive seizures in epileptics.
Warnings: As for all other barbiturates, continued use may lead to habituation. This does not apply to its use in epilepsy. Sudden withdrawal may induce convulsions. Parenteral material should be freshly made up.
Administration: Oral, intramuscular.
Preparations: Tablet, 15 mg., 30 mg., 100 mg. Elixir, 4 mg. per cc. Ampule, 15 mg., 130 mg. Undissolved powder, to be dissolved before using in 1–2 cc. sterile water.
Dose: Depending on use from 15 mg. to 130 mg.
Antidote: Analeptics, such as picrotoxin.

PHENOL—Carbolic Acid
Antiseptic. Light pink crystals with characteristic odor. Solubility with water has important special characteristics. When small amounts of water are mixed with it, a solution of water and phenol is formed which is highly caustic. When large amounts of water are used, the phenol dissolves in the water, forming a far less caustic solution.
Absorption: Rapidly absorbed from G. I. tract.
Actions and Uses: Although freely used years ago, now recognized as relatively

dangerous material for use in or on the patient and is, therefore, not used for antiseptic purposes in medicine. It has great value, however, in decontamination of inanimate objects. In dilute solution (1-2%), it has local anesthetic actions which are made use of in skin preparations. It is sometimes used in highly concentrated form for its caustic properties. Not a dependable general antiseptic. *Warnings*: Highly toxic and caustic. Large amounts can be absorbed from the surface of the skin. May cause central depression. By mouth, it may cause severe burns of the esophagus and stomach.
Administration: Topical.
Preparations: Liquified phenol, 90%. Lotion, 1-2%. Ointment, 1-2%. Glycerite, 5%.
Dose: Concentration varies with indications.
Antidote: Treat with bland oil, topically or by stomach tube as indicated.

PHENOLPHTHALEIN
Cathartic. White to pink varying with the acidity of medium.
Absorption: From G. I. tract.
Actions and Uses: Cathartic, and as with others, continued use may lead to dependence. Commonly used in candy, chewing gum and other forms of "hidden laxatives."
Warnings: May be habit forming. In sensitive individual, small doses have been highly toxic. Relatively frequently causes skin eruptions.
Administration: Oral.
Preparations: Tablet and mixtures with other laxatives.
Dose: 60 mg.

PHENOL RED, see Phenolsulfonphthalein

PHENOLSULFONPHTHALEIN
—Phenol Red
Diagnostic dye. Red powder, slightly soluble in water, more soluble in alkaline solutions.
Actions and Uses: Excreted by kidney and used to determine degree of func-

tional activity of kidney. Its excretion is delayed in the damaged kidney.
Warnings: Intramuscular injection may be painful.
Administration: Intravenous.
Preparations: Ampule, 6 mg. per cc. of the dye in soluble form.
Dose: 6 mg.

PHENOXYBENZAMINE—Dibenzyline®
Adrenolytic.
Actions and Uses: Antagonizes sympathetic and epinephrine constriction of arteries and used in relief of peripheral vasospasm in such conditions as Raynaud's Syndrome, frost bite, thrombophlebitis, etc. and in hypertension of pheochromocytoma.
Warnings: May cause sharp fall in blood pressure. Do not use in anginal syndrome or other forms of coronary artery disease. May cause nausea, headache, drowsiness and malaise.
Administration: Oral.
Preparations: Capsule, 10 mg.
Dose: 10 to 60 mg. daily in divided doses.

PHENOXYMETHYL PENICILLIN
—Penicillin V, Pen-Vee®, V-Cillin®
Another new form of penicillin which is said to be more resistant to destruction by acid and better absorbed from the gastro-intestinal tract than the ordinary penicillin G. Therefore it is recommended for oral use. Also claimed to produce higher and longer lasting blood levels than penicillin G. Available in 200,000-capsules. Dosage the same order as for other forms of penicillin, which see.

PHENSUXIMIDE—Milontin®
Antiepileptic, anticonvulsant.
Actions and Uses: Specifically for the relief of petit mal attacks in epilepsy.
Warnings: Although said to be relatively non-toxic, rashes and drowsiness have been reported.
Administration: Oral.
Preparations: Capsule, 0.5 Gm. Suspension, 250 mg. per teaspoonful.
Dose: 0.5-1.0 Gm. 2-3 times daily.

PHENTETIOTHALEIN—Iso-Iodei-
kon®
Diagnostic. Purple crystals, soluble in
water, the sodium salt.
Actions and Uses: Concentrated in gall-
bladder and used for x-ray of the gall-
bladder and liver function tests.
Warnings: Contraindicated in severe
heart disease and uremia; use carefully
if jaundice is present.
Administration: Intravenous.
Preparations: Ampule, 2.5 Gm.
Dose: 40 mg. per Kg., body weight, but
not exceeding a total of 2.5 Gm.

PHENTOLAMINE—Regitine®
Adrenolytic. White powder, the methane-
sulfonate, hydrochloride or sulfate.
Actions and Uses: Blocks action of the
adrenal medulla, epinephrine and sympathetic stimulation; used to test for
presence of pheochromocytoma, a tumor
of the adrenal.
Warnings: May cause palpitations, hypotension, shock.
Administration: Intramuscular, intravenous, oral.
Preparations: Tablet, 50 mg. Parenteral
solution, ampule containing 5 mg.
Dose: Oral, 50 mg. 3-4 times daily. Parenteral, 5 mg.

PHENURONE®, see Phenacemide

PHENYLAZO-DIAMINO-
PYRIDINE—Pyridium®, Sulfid®
Urinary antiseptic. A yellow orange dye
with antiseptic action which has largely
been superseded in urinary tract infections by more reliable chemotherapeutic
and antibiotic drugs.

PHENYLBUTAZONE—
Butazolidin®
Analgesic. Derivative of aminopyrine
which has recently been introduced with
the claim that it has specific action in
arthritis. Best evidence that its action is
purely one of analgesia. What is of far
more importance, however, is the fact
that, as might have been expected from
our knowledge of the history of aminopyrine, its use has been complicated by

serious and occasionally fatal agranulocytosis.

PHENYLCARBINOL, see Benzyl
Alcohol
PHENYLEPHRINE—Isophrin®,
Neo-Synephrine®
Adrenergic. White crystals with bitter
taste, soluble in water. Usually the hydrochloride.
Actions and Uses: In common with other
members of the sympathomimetic group
of drugs, it is a local vasoconstrictor,
elevating blood pressure, reducing swelling in nasal congestion, and when mixed
with local anesthetics, retards the rate
of absorption. Used in eye as a mydriatic,
in cases in which the use of atropine
seems dangerous. Used in vasomotor collapse.
Warnings: Avoid contact with metal as
much as possible. Store in tightly stoppered bottle and keep out of direct light.
Discard unclear solutions.
Administration: Topical, intravenous, intramuscular, subcutaneous.
Preparations: Parenteral, 10 mg. per cc.,
vial, ampule. Topical, solutions of varying concentration.
Dose: Parenteral, 1-10 mg.

PHENYLHYDRAZINE
Bone marrow depressant which, because
of its toxicity, has been largely replaced
in treatment of polycythemia vera by
acetylphenylhydrazine, which see.

PHENYLMERCURIC NITRATE
—Merphenyl Nitrate®
Organic mercurial antiseptic. White pow-
der, slightly soluble in water.
Actions and Uses: Much as other mem-
bers of the organic mercurial antiseptic
group. Not frequently used at present.
Administration: Topical.
Preparations: Borate as well as nitrate.
Tincture, solution, ointment, mixtures
with picric acid.
Dose: Concentrations 1:500, 1:1500.
Antidote: Dimercaprol.

PHENYLPROPANOLAMINE—Pro-
padrine®
One of the large series of adrenergic

drugs, which see. Used especially for nasal decongestant and vasoconstrictant actions.

PHENYLPROPYLETHYLAMINE —Profenil®

Smooth muscle relaxant. Usefulness remains to be demonstrated. Available in 60 and 120 mg. tablets, and solution for intramuscular administration.

Warnings: May induce hypotension after intramuscular injection.

PHENYLPROPYLMETHYLAMINE —Vonedrine®

One of the large series of adrenergic drugs, which see. Used especially for nasal decongestant action.

PHENYL SALICYLATE—Salol

Pharmaceutic. White powder, barely soluble in water, resistant to acid.

Actions and Uses: Liberates salicylic acid and phenol and was originally used as intestinal antiseptic. Has since been discarded because of danger of toxicity from phenol as well as ineffectiveness as intestinal antiseptic. Its present use is restricted to that of coating pills which, because of resistance to acid, pass untouched through the stomach to the small intestine, the juices of which dissolve off the salol coating.

Warnings: A large number of coated pills may provide enough phenol to cause phenol poisoning in a child.

PHENYLTOLOXAMINE—Histionex®, Bristamin®

Antihistaminic. This drug is a complex of an antihistamine drug with a resin and is said to have a prolonged action, requiring, therefore, only two doses daily for continued action. Dosage of the order of 25 to 50 mg.

PHENYTOIN, see Diphenylhydantoin

pHISODERM with HEXACHLOROPHENE ,see pHisoHex

pHISOHEX—pHisoderm with Hexachlorophene

Antiseptic soap. Creamy liquid which suds when agitated with water.

Actions and Uses: A detergent with cleansing properties with distinct and persistent antibacterial action on the skin. Used to prepare hands and skin for surgery.

Warnings: Store at room temperature. Avoid extremes of temperature.

Administration: As soap.

PHOSPHALGEL®, see Aluminum Phosphate Gel

PHOSPHATE OF SODA, see Sodium Phosphate

PHOSPHORIC ACID

Acidifier. Colorless syrupy liquid, miscible with water.

Absorption: From G. I. tract.

Actions and Uses: Substitute for hydrochloric acid, but since it interferes with the absorption of calcium it is little used today.

PHTHALYLSULFATHIAZOLE —Sulfathalidine®

Chemotherapeutic and sulfonamide. White powder, bitter taste, insoluble in water.

Absorption: Slightly absorbed from G. I. tract (5%).

Actions and Uses: Typical actions of sulfonamides, but not absorbed from intestinal tract, so that high concentration of drug may exert its action throughout the intestinal tract, especially the small bowel and colon. Used in treating inflammatory disease of intestinal tract and in preparing the bowel for surgery. See Sulfonamides.

Warnings: In occasional cases, there may be considerable absorption with the usual dangers of sulfonamides. Though absorption is poor, danger of reaction is present in cases known to be hypersensitive to sulfonamides, hence contraindicated. See Sulfonamides.

Administration: Oral.

Preparations: Tablet, 0.5 Gm.

Dose: 0.05–0.1 Gm. per Kg. body weight, daily, in divided doses.

PHYSOSTIGMINE—Eserine

Cholinergic. White crystals or powder, slightly soluble in water, usually the salicylate.

Actions and Uses: Parasympathetic stim-

ulant action by preventing destruction of acetylcholine, thus permitting it to accumulate and to stimulate the parasympathetic system; same in this respect as neostigmine. Powerful miotic, used to counteract action of atropine. Used to treat abdominal distention in the ileum and also (but usually neostigmine) to treat myasthenia gravis. Used in glaucoma.
Warnings: Overaction may induce violent cramps, depression of blood pressure and convulsions. Solutions should be protected from direct light. Use only clear and colorless solutions.
Administration: Topical and parenteral (rare).
Preparations: Ophthalmic ointment, Ophthalmic solution. Sterile parenteral solution.
Dose: Ophthalmic, 2.5 mg. in each eye. Parenteral, 2 mg.
Antidote: Atropine, 2 mg. intravenously.

PHYTONADIONE—Mephyton®, Vitamin K₁
One of the two naturally occurring forms of Vitamin K with actions said to be somewhat more prolonged than menadione and to be more effective in reversing reactions to overdosage with coumarin drugs. See Menadione.

PICRAGOL®, see Silver Picrate

PICRIC ACID, see Trinitrophenol

PICROTOXIN
Analeptic. Powder or crystals, slightly soluble in water.
Actions and Uses: Convulsant and central stimulant used chiefly in barbiturate poisoning with depressed reflexes.
Warnings: Requires expert supervision and constant attention. Overdosage may produce serious convulsions.
Administration: Intravenous.
Preparations: Vials, 5-10cc., containing 3 mg. per cc.
Dose: Determined by condition of patient.
Antidote: Barbiturates.

PILOCARPINE
Cholinergic. Colorless crystals with bit-

ter taste, soluble in water, usually the hydrochloride.
Actions and Uses: Stimulates many parasympathetic functions by direct action (as compared with the indirect actions of physostigmine). Used to stimulate perspiration, and in ophthalmology as a miotic.
Warnings: In pulmonary disease, the drug may induce pulmonary edema. May cause weakness, excessive perspiration. May induce asthmatic attack. Store away from direct light.
Administration: Topical (ophthalmic), parenteral.
Preparations: Ophthalmic solution, 1 and 2%. Parenteral solution, rarely used.
Dose: Ophthalmic, 1-2 drops in eye. Parenteral, 5 mg.

PINE NEEDLE OIL, DWARF
Inhalant. Yellowish liquid with pleasant characteristic odor.
Actions and Uses: As an inhalant in irritations of respiratory passages.
Dose: 0.3-0.6 cc. in inhaler with steam.

PINE TAR
Antiseptic. Viscid dark brown liquid with characteristic odor.
Actions and Uses: Externally as skin stimulant and antiseptic. Internally (rarely at present) as irritant expectorant.
Warnings: Stains linen. Overdose may markedly irritate respiratory system.
Administration: Topical, oral.
Preparations: Ointment. Expectorant, rarely.
Dose: Concentration, 2–4%.

PIPENZOLATE—Piptal®
Anticholinergic. A new addition to this long list of drugs. Advantages over the others remain to be established. Dosage ranges around 5 mg.

PIPERAT®, see Piperazine

PIPERAZINE—Antepar®, Anthalazine®, Oxucide®, Parazine®, Perin®, Piperat®, Pipzan®, Vermizine®
Vermifuge. Citrate, calcium edathamil, phosphate, gluconate.

Actions and Uses: Recommended for pinworms and roundworms.

Warnings: May cause vomiting; prolonged treatment should be avoided. Weight of children must be taken into account in dosage.

Administration: Oral.

Preparations: Tablet, 250, 500 mg. Syrup, 100 mg. per cc.

Dose: For adults and larger children, 400 mg. twice daily; for infants proportionately smaller doses. Discontinue after 1 week and do not repeat until at least 1 week without medication.

PIPERAZINE ESTRONE SULFATE—Sulestrex Piperazine®

Estrogen. Same actions and uses as naturally occurring conjugated Estrogens, which see.

PIPERIDOLATE—Dactil®

Anticholinergic. New drug; usefulness yet to be established.

PIPEROCAINE—Metycaine®

Surface anesthetic. White crystals or powder soluble in water, bitter taste.

Actions and Uses: Absorbed from mucous membranes and induces local anesthesia by topical application as well as by subcutaneous injection.

Warnings: More toxic than procaine.

Administration: Topical, subcutaneous.

Preparations: Solution, ophthalmic, nasal, parenteral.

Dose: Ophthalmic, 2–4%. Nasal, 2–10%. Infiltration anesthesia, 0.5–1%. Total dose should never exceed 0.75 mg. per pound of body weight and maximum total should not exceed 150 mg.

PIPEROXAN—Benodaine®

Adrenolytic and diagnostic. White crystals, usually the hydrochloride, soluble in water.

Actions and Uses: Antagonizes the action of the adrenal medulla, epinephrine and sympathetic stimulation. A diagnostic for presence of tumor of adrenal, a pheochromocytoma.

Warnings: May cause tachycardia, hypotension, shock.

Administration: Intravenous.

Preparations: Ampule, 10 cc. containing 2 mg.

Dose: 0.25 mg. per Kg. body weight.

PIPRADOL—Meratran®

Stimulant. The hydrochloride.

Actions and Uses: Exerts a cephalotropic action which is not yet definitely localized but apparently in the higher centers. Recommended for mildly depressed patients. Said not to induce "jitters" or to depress appetite. Therapeutic trial has not yet been extensive enough to establish its final position.

Warnings: A new drug; neither toxicity nor potential for habituation have been established. Contraindicated in agitated patients.

Administration: Oral.

Preparations: Tablet, 1 mg.

Dose: 1-2 mg., 2-3 times daily.

PIPTAL®, see Pipenzolate

PIPZAN®, see Piperazine

PITOCIN®, see Oxytocin

PITRESSIN®, see Vasopressin

PITUITARY, POSTERIOR

Hormone. Yellow or gray powder, standardized in U.S.P. Units.

Actions and Uses: Intensifies uterine contraction and is used, therefore, for postpartum hemorrhage and to stimulate prolonged labor. Also stimulates intestinal activity. Antidiuretic in diabetes insipidus. Ineffective orally.

Warnings: Overdosage may cause constriction of gut, spasm of coronary arteries, excessive elevation of blood pressure in patients with hypertension.

Administration: Subcutaneous, intramuscular.

Preparations: Ampule, 1 cc. containing 10 U.S.P. Units "obstetrical" solution.

Dose: Obstetrics, 0.2-1 cc.

PLACEBO

Any preparation administered to satisfy the patient's desire for medication rather than for a pharmacologic action.

PLACIDYL®, see Ethchlorvynol

PLAQUENIL®, see Hydroxychloroquine

PLANTAGO SEED—Psyllium Seed
Laxative.
Actions and Uses: Mucilaginous laxative.
Warnings: Same as for all laxatives regularly used.
Administration: Oral.
Preparations: Dried seed.
Dose: 7.5 Gm.

PLASMA EXPANDERS
Dextran, Gelatin, Hydrodextran, Polyvidone.

PLASMA HYDROLYSATE—Travamin®
A digest of bovine plasma proteins. See Amino Acid Preparations.

PLASMA, NORMAL HUMAN, CITRATED
Parenteral fluid. Plasma from pooled blood from which red cells have been removed and to which citrate has been added to prevent clotting.
Actions and Uses: Replace fluid in blood stream in shock, hemorrhage and other conditions requiring increased blood volume, or blood protein.
Warnings: Examine expiration date. Solution must be filtered while using. Bring to room temperature before using.
Administration: Intravenous.
Preparations: Liquid, frozen and dried.
Dose: 500 cc.

PLASMOCHIN, see Pamaquine

PLASMOQUINE, see Pamaquine

PLAVOLEX®, see Dextran

PLAZMOID®, see Oxypolygelatin

PODOPHYLLUM RESIN SUSPENSION
Skin irritant. Dark brown liquid with characteristic odor. Podophyllum suspended in compound tincture of benzoin.
Actions and Uses: Potent skin irritant, used for treatment of granuloma inguinale and "venereal" warts.
Warnings: Shake well. May be irritating. Avoid normal skin and mucous membranes. Avoid contact with open flame.
Administration: Topical.
Preparations: Suspension.
Dose: Concentration 25%.

POLYAMINE-METHYLENE RESINS—Basex®, ExorbinR, Resinat®, Resion®, Resmicon®
Acid exchange resins.
Actions and Uses: Adsorb and bind hydrochloric acid and inhibit the activity of pepsin. Used in treatment of peptic ulcer. See Exchange resins.
Administration: Oral.
Preparations: Tablet and capsule.
Dose: 1 tablet or capsule every 2 hours.

POLYCYCLINE®, see Tetracycline

POLYESTRADIOL PHOSPHATE—Esradurin®
Estrogen. Recommended especially for carcinoma of the prostate. New drug, special value remains to be established by long clinical trial. Available in 40 mg. ampule with diluent.

POLYETHYLENE GLYCOLS—Carbowax®
Vehicle. A series of materials of different melting points used, in accordance with these properties as a base for water-soluble ointments. The various forms are indicated by their approximate molecular weights thus: 300, 1500, 1540 and 4000.

POLYMYXIN B—Aerosporin®
Antibiotic.
Actions and Uses: New antibiotic with bactericidal properties against gram-negative bacilli and also gram-positive organisms, including staphylococci and streptococci. Used especially against *Pseudomonas aeruginosa* (*B. pyocyaneus*) infections, including septicemia, meningitis, urinary tract infections, middle ear infections, liver abscess, severe burns and certain infections of the respiratory tract and the joints.
Warnings: Should be used parenterally only under close medical supervision. When administered topically in the ear, external canal should be cleaned and dried thoroughly before application.
Administration: Topical, intramuscular.
Preparations: Vial, 500,000 Units (50 mg.). Solution.
Dose: 50 mg.

POLYSORB
Pharmaceutic. Used in the preparation of hydrophilic ointments.

POLYSORBATE 80—Sorbitan
Emulsifier.

POLYVIDONE — PVP-Macrose®,
Vinisil®
Plasma expander. Solution containing, in addition to electrolyte, synthetic macromolecules which exert osmotic tension and have hydrophilic properties.
Actions and Uses: Used as a substitute to whole blood and plasma in the same situations in which the former are indicated, especially when they are not readily available or, for one reason or another, cannot be used. Saves time since requires no typing.
Warnings: Although untoward effects are not reported, this material has not the benefit of wide-scale testing and should be used only in instances in which whole blood or plasma are not available. Inject slowly.
Administration: Intravenous.
Preparations: Solution, 3.5%, with electrolyte.
Dose: As indicated by condition.

PONTOCAINE®, see Tetracaine

POQUIL®, see Pyrrovinylquinium

POSTERIOR PITUITARY, see
Pituitary, Posterior

POTASSIC SALINE—Darrow's
Solution
Electrolyte. A clear parenteral saline solution containing potassium.
Actions and Uses: In the treatment of dehydration and acidosis associated with potassium deficiency, especially after severe diarrhea.
Warnings: The possibility of hyperpotassemia must be considered while using this solution. Slow administration and frequent examination of the blood for potassium and the electrocardiogram for cardiac signs of hyperpotassemia are essential.
Administration: Subcutaneous, rarely intravenous.

Preparations: Ampules, 500 cc.
Dose: Not to exceed 80 cc. per Kg. in 12 hours.

POTASSIUM ACETATE
Alkali. White powder or crystalline material with saline taste, soluble in water.
Actions and Uses: Systemic alkali and diuretic, similar to sodium acetate.
Warnings: Administered in milk or water.
Administration: Oral.
Preparations: Powder and crystals.
Dose: 1 Gm.

POTASSIUM AMINOSALICYLATE
—Paskalium®, Paskate®
Potassium salt of Aminosalicylic Acid. Used in tuberculosis, usually in conjunction with other antituberculars. See Para-Aminosalicylic Acid.

POTASSIUM ARSENITE—
Fowler's Solution
Hematinic and arsenical. White powder, soluble in water.
Actions and Uses: A hematinic used at present as temporary medication with benefit in chronic myelogenous leukemia. Used also in certain skin lesions.
Warnings: Toxicity of arsenic is high.
Administration: Oral.
Preparations: Solution, Fowler's solution (1%).
Dose: 0.1 to 0.3 cc. daily until toxic signs appear. Dose may be increased steadily by small increments, if indicated.
Antidote: Dimercaprol.

POTASSIUM BICARBONATE
Alkali. White powder, soluble in water.
Actions and Uses: A mild alkali ordinarily with no advantages over the much less expensive sodium bicarbonate. However, in cases in which sodium is contraindicated, potassium bicarbonate may be substituted.
Warnings: Overdosage may lead to potassium intoxication.
Administration: Oral.
Preparations: Solution and tablet.
Dose: 1 Gm., or as indicated.

POTASSIUM BROMIDE
Bromide sedative.
Actions and Uses: Has no special ad-

vantages, but all the disadvantages of bromides and, as with them, little place in modern medicine.
Antidote: Sodium chloride.

POTASSIUM CHLORATE
Oxidant. Highly active chemical. Use in medicine is questionable at best.
Warnings: Large doses may be poisonous and cause blood dyscrasias.

POTASSIUM CHLORIDE
Electrolyte. White powder, soluble in water with saline taste.
Actions and Uses: Source of the potassium ion for electrolyte in fluids. Potassium normally is present in small amounts in body fluids; used to replace this in cases in which it is low. Has diuretic action. Used sometimes as a salt substitute.
Warnings: Potassium salts given in large doses, or in case of renal insufficiency, may cause potassium intoxication.
Administration: Oral, intravenously in parenteral fluids.
Preparations: Tablet. Solution, in Ringer's solution, as concentrate to be added to infusion fluids when needed.
Dose: Oral, 1 Gm. Intravenous, as indicated by state of electrolyte imbalance.

POTASSIUM CITRATE
Alkali. White powder, soluble in water.
Actions and Uses: Alkali, used systemically; in common with other potassium salts, a diuretic. Use decreasing.
Warnings: Overdose, or use in kindey insufficiency may lead to potassium intoxication.
Administration: Oral.
Preparations: Solution and effervescent powder.
Dose: 1 Gm.

POTASSIUM IODIDE—KI
Expectorant and antifungal. Colorless crystals, soluble in water.
Actions and Uses: As other iodides. Also a saline expectorant and a specific in syphilis for absorption of connective tissue lesions (gummae). Also of value in actinomycosis, sporotrichosis, and blastomycosis.

Warnings: As for iodides and potassium salts.
Administration: Oral.
Preparations: Solution, saturated. Tablet.
Dose: Solution, 0.3 cc. to 2.0 cc. depending on indication. Tablet, 0.3 Gm.

POTASSIUM NITRATE
Diuretic. Transparent crystals or white powder, odorless.
Actions and Uses: An obsolete diuretic.
Warnings: May be highly irritant to intestine and kidneys.
Administration: Oral.
Dose: 1 Gm.

POTASSIUM PENICILLIN, see Penicillin

POTASSIUM PENICILLIN O—Cer-O-Cillin®
Antibiotic. Said to be less allergenic than Penicillin G.

POTASSIUM PERMANGANATE
Antiseptic. Dark purple crystals, soluble in water.
Actions and Uses: An actively oxidizing chemical exerting antiseptic actions. Also used for this action to cleanse wounds and to destroy drugs taken in overdosage, accidentally or deliberately; used as an oxidant to destroy snake venom in snake bites.
Warnings: Highly toxic and active chemical. Solutions must not exceed indicated concentration. When used as antidote to alkaloidal poisoning, care must be taken (in the urgency) not to make solution too strong or it will cause irreparable damage to stomach. Stains linens. Solution turns brown in color during oxidation. Store solutions in containers protected from light.
Administration: Topical, oral (in drug poisoning).
Preparations: Solution, stock (3%), dilutions of 1:500 to 1:10,000. Tablet, 65 mg., 130 mg., 200 mg., 300 mg.
Dose: Concentration as indicated.

POTASSIUM SODIUM TAR-TRATE—Rochelle Salt
Saline cathartic. White powder with saline taste, soluble in water.

Actions and Uses: Mild saline cathartic.
Warnings: In common with all the cathartics, continued use leads to dependence.
Store in tightly stoppered containers.
Administration: Oral.
Preparations: Compound effervescent powders (Seidlitz).
Dose: 10 Gm.

POTASSIUM THIOCYANATE
Hypotensive. Effectiveness is in question. Use is cumbersome; to be carefully followed with blood tests. Overdosage may lead to serious intoxication and blood dyscrasias. Blood levels must be followed for safe use. Little used in scientific medicine. See Thiocyanates.

POVIDONE-IODINE—Betadine®, Isodine®
Local antiseptic. Organic iodide said to
Local antiseptic. Organic iodine said to be more effective and less irritant than Tr. Iodine. Used in 0.5, 0.2 and 0.5% dilutions.

PRAMOXINE—Tronothane®
Surface anesthetic, which see. The hydrochloride. Administered topically, usually in a 1% lotion, solution, cream, or jelly.

PRANONE®, see Ethisterone

PRANTAL®, see Diphemanil

PRECIPITATED CHALK, see Calcium Carbonate

PRECIPITATED SULFUR, see Sulfur

PREDNISOLONE—Delta-Cortef®, Hydeltra®, Meticortelone®, Paracortol®, Sterane®
Anti-inflammatory hormone. A hydrocortisone derivative which is both more potent and less toxic than hydrocortisone. Recent evidence indicates that it can be used without difficulty for longer periods of time than cortisone and hydrocortisone, hence is usually preferable. In general, however, the indications and the precautions to be taken are the same. Available in 2.5 and 5 mg. tablets.

PREDNISONE — Deltasone®, Deltra®, Meticorten®, Paracort®
Anti-inflammatory hormone. A cortisone derivative which has considerably greater potency than cortisone with appreciably less of the undesirable effects. In its use, the indications are generally much the same as with cortisone, and the precautions are also the same. Available in 5 mg. tablets.

PRELUDIN®, see Phenmetrazine

PREMARIN®, see Estrogenic Substances, Conjugated

PREPARED NEOCALAMINE, see Neocalamine

PRIMAQUINE
Antimalarial. Dosage of the order of 15 mg.

PRIMIDONE—Mysoline®
Anticonvulsant. Reduced barbiturate.
Actions and Uses: Anticonvulsant action exerted in all forms of epilepsy.
Warnings: A new drug which requires further trial. Blood should be examined regularly and kidney and liver function observed.
Administration: Oral.
Preparations: Tablet, 0.25 Gm.
Dose: 0.25 Gm. daily.

PRIODAX®, see Iodoalphionic Acid

PRISCOLINE®, see Tolazoline

PRIVINE®, see Naphazoline

PRO-BANTHINE®, see Propantheline

PROBARBITAL—Ipral®
One of the intermediate acting barbiturates, which see.

PROBENECID—Benemid®
Uricosuric. Synthetic, stable, slightly soluble in water, nearly tasteless.
Actions and Uses: Diminishes uric acid content of blood and increases urinary excretion of uric acid 30-50%. Used in the treatment of gout and chronic gouty arthritis, also to intensify action of penicillin and other drugs by retarding excretion in urine.
Warnings: Salicylates should not be administered concurrently because of an antagonism between the two drugs.
Administration: Oral.
Preparations: Tablet, 0.5 Gm.

Dose: 0.5 Gm. daily for 1 week, then 1 Gm. daily in divided doses.

PROBUTYLIN®, see Procaine Isobutyrate

PROCAINE—Novocain®
Local anesthetic. White powder, in form of salts such as hydrochloride or borate, rapidly soluble in water.
Absorption: Not absorbed from surface of skin or mucous membranes.
Actions and Uses: An effective local anesthetic, which is far less toxic, and hence, probably safer than cocaine and other local anesthetics. It has disadvantage of not being effective by topical application, hence not useful in surface anesthesia. For regional and local anesthesia, it is injected into areas in which it is used, but because of the rapidity with which it is destroyed in the body, often it is given together with small amounts of epinephrine, or other vasoconstrictor, to delay its absorption into the bloodstream. It is also used by intravenous injection for special effects such as relieving diffuse itching and generalized allergic reactions. Used for spinal anesthesia. Procaine, but especially its amide is of value in the treatment of disturbances of cardiac rhythm.
Warnings: Overdosage may cause convulsions and death. Reduces blood pressure, and may cause respiratory failure.
Administration: Subcutaneous, intramuscular, intrathecal, intravenous.
Preparations: Solution, sterile, with many special mixtures, especially in the case of materials for dental surgery.
Dose: Regional anesthesia, 0.5–2.0%. Spinal anesthesia, 1.5%. Intravenous, 0.5%. Total dose should not exceed 2 Gm. in 24 hours.
Antidote: Barbiturates.

PROCAINE AMIDE—Pronestyl®
Cardiac depressant. White crystals, soluble in water.
Absorption: From G. I. tract.
Actions and Uses: Effects on heart are much like quinidine. Used in treatment of cardiac arrhythmias, especially those of ventricular origin. Said not to be as

effective in auricular arrhythmias. Chief advantage over quinidine is intravenous administration. Action is same as that of procaine, but of longer duration and permits oral administration. Effects develop immediately after intravenous administration, in about 30 minutes after oral administration.
Warnings: Sharp fall in blood pressure may follow intravenous injection. Not recommended for prophylactic use. Intravenous injections must be made slowly.
Preparations: Capsule, 0.25 Gm. Ampule, 10 cc., 100 mg. per cc.
Dose: Oral, 1.0 Gm., followed by 0.5–1.0 Gm. every 4–6 hours. Intravenous, 2–10 cc. (200 mg. to 1.0 Gm.) slowly, not exceeding 2 cc. per minute.

PROCAINE ISOBUTYRATE—Probutylin®
Local anesthetic. A new drug introduced with claims of useful action in the relief of nausea, vomiting, pylorospasm. Whether it exerts a local action which provides better relief than some of the other new agents now available remains to be established. Possesses the dangers of procaine and should not be used in patients with hypertension.
Preparations: Capsule, 300 mg.
Dose: Of the order of 300-600 mg.

PROCAINE PENICILLIN, see Penicillin

PROCLORPERAZINE—Compazine®
Tranquilizer. New drug, closely related to chlorpromazine. Final position as a tranquilizer remains to be established. Available in 5 mg. tablets.

PROCYCLIDINE—Kemadrin®
Skeletal muscle relaxant. An anticholinergic drug recommended for parkinsonism. Advantages over similar drugs for the same condition remain to be established. Dosage of the order of 2.5 mg. three times a day.

PROFENIL®, see Phenylpropylethylamine

PROGESTERONE—Colprosterone®, Corlutone®, Lucorteum®,

PROGESTIN

Lutocylin®, Lutromone®, Pro-
gestin®, Proluton®, Syngeste-
rone®
Hormone. White powder, insoluble in
water.
Absorption: Not absorbed, from G. I.
tract.
Actions and Uses: Derived from corpus
luteum of the ovary, and is essential for
the implantation of the fertilized egg in
the uterus and the maintenance of pregnancy. Used in cases of habitual spon-
taneous abortion.
Warnings: Quickly destroyed in the body;
to maintain effects dose should be given
at relatively frequent intervals for about
48 hours. Large doses may cause headache. Not administered intravenously.
Administration: Intramuscular. For oral
preparation, see Ethisterone, U.S.P.
Preparations: Ampule, 10–20 mg. per cc.
in oil.
Dose: 5–30 mg.

PROGESTIN®, see Progesterone
PROGUANIL, see Chloroguanide
PROGYNON®, see Estradiol
PROLAX®, see Mephenesin
PROLUTON®, see Progesterone
PROMAZINE—Sparine®
Tranquilizer. Very closely related to
Chlorpromazine. A new drug with which
considerable experience is needed to
establish differences between its uses and
dangers and those of Chlorpromazine,
which see.

**PROMETHAZINE—Fargan®, Phe-
nergan®**
One of the large series of antihistamine
drugs, which see. Also effective against
pin worms after a large single dosage
(125 mg.).

PROMETHESTROL—Meprane®
Synthetic estrogen.
Actions and Uses: Much as diethylstil-
bestrol, which see.

PROMIN®, see Glucosulfone
PROMIZOLE®, see Thiazolsulfone
PROMOXOLANE—Dimethylane®
A very recently introduced drug with a

depressant action on spinal inter-neural
connections which, it is claimed, relieves
tension and spasm by this action but
without central depression. Also suggested for dysmenorrhea and the menopausal syndrome. Considerably more trial
is essential for a well formulated opinion
on the value of this drug.

PRONESTYL®, see Procaine
Amide
PROPADRINE®, see Phenylpro-
panolamine
**PROPANTHELINE—Pro-
Banthine®**
Anticholinergic.
Actions and Uses: Much the same as
methantheline over which it has the ad-
vantage of taste. Other advantages are to
be determined. See methantheline, also
for warnings.

PROPASA®, see Para-Aminosalicylic Acid
**PROPIONATE COMPOUND — Pro-
pion Gel®**
A mixture of the calcium and sodium
propionates used as an antifungal agent.
See Propionic Acid.

PROPION GEL®, see Propionic
Acid
PROPIONIC ACID
Antifungal. The calcium salt, a white
powder soluble in water; the acid a
colorless liquid miscible in water.
Actions and Uses: Antifungal, much the
same as caprylic acid and undecylenic
acid. Usually used in mixtures containing other antifungal agents.

PROPYLENE GLYCOL
Solvent. Colorless viscid liquid, miscible
with water, with little taste.
Actions and Uses: Relatively nontoxic
material used for pharmaceutical preparations in drugs which present special
problems in dissolving.

**PROPYLHEXEDRINE—Benze-
drex®**
Adrenergic and nasal decongestant.
Volatile.
Absorption: Absorbed from nasal mu-
cosa.

Actions and Uses: Much the same as amphetamine but has much less of the pressor action, hence more satisfactory for nasal decongestion which is its only use.
Warnings: In rare instances may elevate blood pressure or irritate nasal mucosa. Discard inhaler after 2–3 months.
Administration: Inhalation.
Preparations: Inhaler containing 0.25 mg.
Dose: Two inhalations in each nostril.

PROPYLIODINE—Dionosil®
Diagnostic. New radio-opaque iodide used for bronchography.

PROPYLPARABEN
Pharmaceutic. Used in the preparation of hydrophilic ointment.

PROPYLTHIOURACIL
Thyroid depressant. White powder, slightly soluble in water, bitter taste.
Actions and Uses: Depresses formation of thyroid hormone (thyroxin) by the thyroid gland. Used in treatment of hyperthyroidism (thyrotoxicosis). In some instances no other medication may be necessary; in others, the use of iodine is helpful. But in most cases, despite the effectiveness of the drug, surgery should be contemplated. The latter course is especially practical because drug requires constant attention. In general, it gives far better results than obtained with iodine alone.
Warnings: Overdose may lead to hypothyroidism, enlargement of thyroid gland, and may lead to increase in vascularity of the gland, making surgery difficult. In hypersensitive cases, blood dyscrasias may develop (more common with older preparation, now discarded, thiouracil) and blood counts should be taken regularly. Look for sore throat, fever, coryza and malaise as early symptoms of granulocytopenia. Discontinue medication if any such symptoms appear.
Administration: Oral.
Preparations: Tablet, 25 mg., 50 mg.
Dose: Depending on severity of case; average about 100 mg. daily in divided doses.

PROSTIGMIN®, see Neostigmine
PROTAMIDE®
Colloidal solution of denatured proteolytic enzymes from hog stomach. Recommended for a variety of neuralgic pains often resistant to treatment by standard measures, herpes zoster, tabetic pains, etc. Substantial evidence for its therapeutic value as well as a reasonable explanation for its reported success are wanting.

PROTAMINE ZINC INSULIN,
see Insulin
PROTARGIN®, see Silver Protein
PROTECTIVES
Demulcents, Collodion, Covicone®.

PROTEIN CONCENTRATE—
Protinal®
Nutritional. Derived from milk, fairly palatable and may be used as a food supplement in cases in which a high protein diet is desirable. It is virtually sodium free. Usually mixed with other foods in the diet.

PROTEIN HYDROLYSATE
—Amino Acid Preparations
Nutritional.
Actions and Uses: Materials derived from milk or animal proteins which, by one form of chemical reaction or another, are reduced to simpler forms. Soluble and may be more readily available for utilization in instances in which there is difficulty in digestion, absorption, assimilation or utilization of food proteins. The mixtures are such that the proper amounts of all essential amino acids are present and the hydrolysates are, in that sense, complete proteins. Since they are soluble, they may be given by parenteral as well as the oral route.
Warnings: Intravenous injection may cause systemic reactions: fever, flush, hypotension, cramps, convulsions. Never add medicaments to an infusion. Reject unclear solutions.
Administration: Oral, intravenous.
Preparations: There is a large variety of these materials, many with little differences. There are some which have special value because they are sodium free. All

come already in solution if they are for intravenous use. There are also many oral preparations, many with particularly bad tastes, though some are well flavored.

PROTEIN PREPARATIONS
Amino acid mixtures, Aminopeptodrate Plasma hydrolysate, Protein hydrolysate, Protein concentrates.

PROTHROMADIN®, see Warfarin

PROTINAL®, see Protein Concentrate

PROTOLYSATE®, see Amino Acid Preparations

PROTOVERATRINES A and B— Provell®, Veralba®
Extracts from Veratrum alba of unknown structure. Said to induce vasodilatation and recommended for treatment of essential hypertension because of this action. There are many toxic side-effects and considerably more experience is required with this drug before its position in the therapy of hypertension is established.

PROVELL®, see Proveratines A and B

PRO-VITAMIN A, see Carotene

P.S.P. DYE, see Phenolsulfonphthalein

PSYLLIUM SEED, see Plantago Seed

PUMICE
Abrasive and absorbent. Light, hard porous powder, insoluble in water.
Actions and Uses: Used in pharmaceutical field as an abrasive and an absorbent.

PURGATIVES, see Cathartics

PURINETHOL®, see Mercaptopurine

PURODIGIN®, see Digitoxin

PVP-MACROSE, see Polyvidone

PYKOTANIN®, see Methylrosaniline

PYRAMAL®, see Pyrilamine

PYRA-MALEATE®, see Pyrilamine

PYRAMIDON®, see Aminopyrine

PYRATHIAZINE—Pyrrolazote®
Antihistaminic. Another of this long series of drugs, which see. Agranulocytosis has been reported following its use. Usual dose of the order of 25 to 100 mg.

PYRETHRUM
Insecticide. Orange powder.
Actions and Uses: A contact poison for many insects; frequently found in the home in commercial insecticides, usually in solution in kerosene. Sometimes applied to the skin in cases of scabies.
Warnings: Frequently causes dermatitis.
Administration: Topical.
Preparations: Ointment.
Dose: Concentration, 0.75%.

PYRIBENZAMINE®, see Tripelennamine

PYRIDIUM®, see Phenylazodiamino-pyridine

PYRIDOSTIGMIN—Mestinon®
Cholinergic. Cholinesterase inhibitor which results in vagal stimulation. Recommended for myesthenia gravis. Advantages over Prostigmine remain to be established. Dosage of the order of 10-60 mg. tablets daily, although many more and occasionally many less may be required.

PYRIDOXINE—Vitamin B$_6$
Nutritional. White powder, soluble in water, the hydrochloride.
Actions and Uses: Aside from its probable essential nutritional nature, it has limited and unproven value in medicine. Recommended for nausea of pregnancy and radiation sickness.
Administration: Oral, parenteral.
Preparations: Tablet: 25 and 50 mg. Solution, 50 mg. in 10 cc.
Dose: Neither the daily requirements nor medical dosages have been determined with any certainty; said to be about the same as that of thiamin.

PYRILAMINE—Copsamine®, Neo-Antergen®, Paraminyl®, Pyramal®, Pyra-Maleate®, Stangen®, Statomin®, Thylogen®
One of the large series of antihistamine drugs, which see.

PYRIMETHAMINE—Daraprim®
Antimalarial. A new agent whose dangers and uses remain to be established.

PYRIZIDIN®, see Isoniazid

PYROGALLIC ACID, see Pyrogallol

PYROGALLOL—Pyrogallic Acid
Irritant skin antiseptic. White needles, changing to brown on exposure to air. Soluble in water.
Absorption: From G. I. tract.
Actions and Uses: In chronic skin diseases as a skin antiseptic.
Warnings: Highly toxic internally. Do not apply over large areas of skin.
Administration: Topical.
Preparations: Ointment.
Dose: Concentration, 2-10%.

PYRONIL®, see Pyrrobutamine

PYROXYLIN—Soluble Guncotton Base.
Actions and Uses: Dissolved in ether and alcohol to form collodion. Used to form a protective film for external medicaments.

PYRROBUTAMINE—Pyronil®
One of the large series of antihistamine drugs, which see.

PYRROLAZOTE®, see Pyrathiazine

PYRROVINYLQUINIUM—Poquil®
Vermifuge. Used in oxyuriasis. Available in suspension.

PYRVINIUM—Vanquin®
Vermifuge. Recommended especially for oxyuriasis. New drug; value yet to be established.

Q

QUASSIA
Vermifuge. Yellow powder with bitter taste.
Actions and Uses: Used in enema in treatment of pin worms.
Administration: Oral, rectal.
Preparations: Solution.
Dose: 0.5 Gm.

QUELICIN®, see Succinylcholine

QUINACRINE—Atabrine®, Mepacrine®
Antimalarial. Bright yellow powder with a bitter taste. Soluble in water.
Actions and Uses: Destroys asexual forms of malarial parasite. About as effective as quinine, but somewhat less toxic. Usually suppressive and cures only falciparum form of malaria.
Warnings: Causes yellow discoloration of skin, sclera and urine. May cause G. I. distress, dermatitis, rarely delirium, hepatitis, aplastic anemia.
Administration: Oral (preferable), intravenous, intramuscular.
Preparations: Tablet, 0.1 Gm. Ampule, 0.2 Gm. of drug to be dissolved in 5 cc. water before using.
Dose: Oral, depending on whether for treatment or for prophylaxis (suppressive). Single dose 0.1-0.2 Gm. Schedules vary. Intramuscular, 0.4 Gm., half in one buttock and half in the other. Repeat if necessary.

QUINIDINE
Cardiac depressant. The sulfate is white powder, soluble in water, has bitter taste.
Absorption: Rapidly absorbed from G. I. tract.
Actions and Uses: Has the same actions and potency as quinine in malaria, but rarely used for that purpose, largely because of its cost. May be used instead of quinine in cases sensitive to the latter. Used in cardiac arrhythmias of all types, in which it is far superior to quinine.
Warnings: May cause cinchonism (nausea, ringing in ears, dizziness) as well as diarrhea, sweating, flushing, apprehension, skin rash, urticaria. Test dose often given. Intravenous use is dangerous.
Administration: Oral (preferable), intramuscular, intravenous (dangerous).
Preparations: Tablet, 0.2 Gm., 0.3 Gm. Ampule, solution on the market for parenteral use. Discard any of the latter which is discolored. Some solutions contain aminopyrine, and should not be used in cases of aminopyrine sensitivity.
Dose: Oral, 0.3 Gm. every 3-4 hours, or

more if necessary, since it is rapidly excreted. Intramuscular, as oral.

QUININE

Antimalarial. White powder; solubility depends on chemical form. Bitter taste. As sulfate, dihydrochloride, bisulfate, hydrobromide, hydrochloride, phosphate.
Absorption: From G. I. tract.
Actions and Uses: The oldest specific remedy in medicine. Has cardiac actions of quinidine, but not as potent and rarely used for this purpose. Has analgesic and antipyretic actions, for which it is sometimes found in headache remedies, etc., usually, however, in small amounts because it is so much more expensive than other analgesics. An effective remedy for malaria, but giving way to the more effective ones now available.
Warnings: Intravenous use may cause serious reactions. Cinchonism (ringing in the ears, nausea, dizziness) is common. Also may cause urticaria, skin rashes, blackwater fever, abortion in late pregnancy, deafness, convulsions, collapse. May prolong prothrombin time.
Administration: Oral (preferable), intravenous (in emergencies).
Preparations: Tablet, capsule, 0.2-0.3 Gm. Solution, for children. Parenteral solution, the dihydrochloride is usually used.
Dose: Depends on use, whether treatment or prophylactic (suppressive). Oral, 0.5-1.0 Gm. in single doses. Intravenous, 0.5 Gm.

QUININE AND UREA HYDRO-CHLORIDE

Sclerotic. Colorless crystals or white powder, soluble in water.
Actions and Uses: Although this may be used as a parenteral material in malaria, its main use is as a sclerotic agent in the treatment of varicose veins and hemorrhoids. It also has a local anesthetic action which, at one time was widely made use of, but has since given way to more effective and less irritant materials.
Warnings: As for quinine, with additional fact that it is highly irritant and may cause local necrosis. Protect from light.

Administration: Intravenous.
Preparations: Ampule, 100 mg. in 2 cc.
Dose: Sclerosing agent, 1-2 cc.

QUININE CARBACRYLIC RESIN —Diagnex®

Exchange resin: Used in test for gastric acidity without gastric intubation.

QUOTANE®, see Dimethisoquin

R

RABELLON®, see Belladonna

RACEMORPHAN — Dromoran®, Methorphinan

Addictive analgesic.
Actions and Uses: Highly potent analgesic. More potent and longer acting than morphine. Used in relieving serious pain. See Morphine.
Warnings: Respiratory depression is about the same as that caused by morphine. Narcotic and under the control of federal narcotic laws.
Administration: Subcutaneous.
Preparations: Ampule, 5 mg. per cc. Vial, 10 cc., 5 mg. per cc.
Dose: 2.5-5 mg.
Antidote: Nalorphine.

RACEPHEDRINE—I-sedrine®, see Ephedrine

RADIOACTIVE METALS

Radiocobalt, Radiochromate, Radio gold, Radioiodine, Radiophosphorus.

RADIOCOBALT

Anticarcinogenic. A radioactive isotope used in the treatment of certain forms of carcinoma.

RADIO-CHROMATE SODIUM— Cr^{51}

Diagnostic. Used as a biologic tracer mainly to determine blood volume, red cell volume, and red cell survival time.

RADIO-GOLD COLLOID—Au^{198}

Radioactive gold is recommended for the irradiation of serious cavities in the palliative treatment of effusions due to carcinomatosis.

RADIOIODINE—I¹³¹
Anticarcinogenic and antithyroid. A radioactive isotope of iodine which is concentrated in thyroid gland after oral administration and which exerts the effects of radiation in that area. Used in the treatment of hyperthyroidism and in a few instances of carcinoma of the thyroid.

RADIOPHOSPHATE SODIUM—P³²
Anticarcinogenic. A radioactive isotope of phosphorus which tends to a certain degree to concentrate in the bone marrow; used, in certain types of leukemia.

RAMETIN®, see Vitamin B_{12}

RAPACODIN®, see Dihydrocodeine

RAPHETAMINE®, see Amphetamine

RASPBERRY
Flavor. Juice of the fruit with characteristic taste and odor.
Actions and Uses: As a flavor.
Preparations: Syrup.

RAUDIXIN®, see Rauwolfia

RAURINE®, see Reserpine

RAU-SED®, see Reserpine

RAU-TAB®, see Alseroxylon

RAUWILOID®, see Alseroxylon

RAUWISTAN®, see Rauwolfia

RAUWOLFIA
Hypotensive, sedative.
This drug in a variety of crude, partially purified and crystalline forms has recently been introduced on the market with claims for great utility in the treatment of essential hypertension. In addition it is also sold in mixtures with extract of Veratrum, with Hydralazine and even hexamethonium. A specific action on blood vessels in hypertension is yet to be demonstrated. Proof is lacking, therefore, that Rauwolfia in any of its forms contributes anything to the patient with hypertension, beyond sedation. A central depressant action has been demonstrated and this is, perhaps, its most certain effect, providing mild sedation with small doses and, in larger doses, sedating intense anxiety and excitement of neuroses and psychoses. At present the latter probably constitutes the largest use of this drug. No important difference between the various extracts has been demonstrated. The dangers of this material have not yet been fully established. Stuffiness of the nose is common. Parkinsonism and psychotic reactions have also been reported.
Whole root. Mixture of alkaloids; Alseroxylon. *Purified alkaloids;* Deserpedine, Rescinnamine, Reserpine.

RECTIFIED TAR OIL
Parasiticide. Thin liquid with brown color and characteristic odor. Insoluble in water.
Actions and Uses: Occasionally used for expectorant, usually externally in skin diseases.
Warnings: Stains linens. Prolonged use is dangerous.
Administration: Oral, topical.
Preparations: Syrup, 0.1%. Ointment, 1–4%.
Dose: Oral, 10 cc.

RECTIFIED TURPENTINE OIL, see Turpentine Oil

RED BLOOD CELLS, see Blood, Whole (Packed Cells)

REDISOL®, see Vitamin B_{12}

REGITINE®, see Phentolamine

RELAXIN—Releasin®
Hormone. A new hormone said to cause relaxation of publis during pregnancy. Recommended to diminish intensity and diminish frequency of uterine contractions and halt premature labor. Utility remains to be established. Available in 20 mg. ampules. The usual dose of 1 cc. every 4 hours by muscle or in an intravenous drip.

RELEASIN®, see Relaxin

RENIN
Digestive enzyme. Yellowish powder, partially soluble in water.
Actions and Uses: Used for making

whey, junket and to coagulate milk protein.

REPETAB
Proprietary name for a tablet which is so prepared as to confer an unusually prolonged action on any drug incorporated in it.

RESCINNAMINE—Moderil®
Tranquilizer. Rauwolfia material, which see. No evidence that it differs materially from other highly purified rauwolfia materials. Usefulness can only be established after long clinical trial. Also used in hypertension. Available in 0.25 and 0.5 mg. tablets.

RESERPINE—Crystoserpine® Raurine®, Rau-Sed®, Reserpoid®, Sandril®, Serfin®, Serpasil®, Serpiloid®
A pure form of alkaloid from Rauwolfia. Available in 0.1-1.0 mg. tablets, and 5 mg. vials. Dosage 0.1-1.0 mg. daily. *Warnings:* The incidence of reactions is relatively high when dosage exceeds 0.3 mg. daily.

RESERPOID®, see Reserpine

RESINAT®, see Polyamine-methylene Resins

RESINS, see Exchange resins

RESION®, see Polyamine-methylene Resins

RESMICON®, see Polyamine-methylene Resins

RESODEC®, see Carboxylic Resins

RESORCIN, see Resorcinol

RESORCINOL—Resorcin.
Antiseptic. White crystals, soluble in water.
Actions and Uses: Used as a skin irritant and antiseptic in skin diseases.
Warnings: Turns light hair dark. Store in dark. Highly toxic when taken internally. For external use only. Skin sensitization occurs.
Administration: Topical.
Preparations: Lotion.
Dose: Concentration, 1-4%.

RESPIRATORY STIMULANTS
Aminophylline, Ammonia, Caffeine, Carbon dioxide, Lobeline, Nikethamide Oxygen, Pentylenetetrazol, Picrotoxin.

RESTROL®, see Dienestrol

RHUBARB
Cathartic. Orange powder.
Actions and Uses: Laxative.
Warnings: Same as for all laxatives, in that continued use tends to habituation.
Administration: Oral.
Preparations: There is a host of preparations, none with great virtue over any other: alkaline rhubarb elixir, rhubarb extract, rhubarb fluidextract, compound rhubarb powder, rhubarb and soda mixture, rhubarb syrup, aromatic rhubarb syrup, rhubarb tincture, aromatic rhubarb tincture, sweet rhubarb tincture.
Dose: The equivalent of 0.5-2.0 Gm. of the powder.

RIBOFLAVIN—Vitamin B$_2$, Lactoflavin
Vitamin. Orange powder, slightly soluble in water.
Absorption: From G. I. tract.
Actions and Uses: Provides needed vitamin in cases of riboflavin deficiency. This may exist in a nearly pure form of vitamin deficiency or together with other deficiencies, in which case, other vitamins may be necessary. Because pure deficiencies rarely exist, it is usually used together with other vitamins. A nontoxic material.
Warnings: Protect from light.
Administration: Oral, parenteral.
Preparations: Capsule, 1 mg., 2 mg., 5 mg. Ampule, sterile solution containing 5 mg. riboflavin and a stabilizer, to be dissolved in 2-3 cc. water before using. Mixture, with other vitamins.
Dose: Oral and parenteral, 2-15 mg. daily.

RIMIFON®, see Isoniazid

RINGER'S SOLUTION
Parenteral fluid. A clear colorless solution containing physiologic concentrations of sodium chloride, calcium chloride, potassium chloride.

Actions and Uses: Same as for isotonic saline, but contains calcium and potassium and therefore less likely to cause electrolyte disturbances. Also used in cases in which there is potassium deficiency.
Warnings: Rapid injection, especially in the cardiac patient, may cause serious reactions.
Administration: Intravenous, subcutaneous.
Dose: As indicated by circumstances.

RITALIN®, see Methylphenidate

ROBALATE®, see Dihydroxyaluminum Aminoacetate

ROBAXIN®, see Methocarbamol

ROCHELLE SALT, see Potassium Sodium Tartrate

ROLICTON®, see Aminoisometradine

ROMILAR®, see Dextromethorphan

RONIACOL®, see Beta-pyridyl carbinol

ROSEMARY OIL
Flavor.
Actions and Uses: Aromatic oil for flavoring. Also carminative and rubefacient.

ROSE OIL
Perfume.
Preparations: Rose water, rose water ointment.

ROSIN
Base, rubefacient.
Actions and Uses: Used in preparation of ointments and plasters; also as a rubefacient.

ROTENONE
Parasiticide. An insecticide used commonly in the spraying and dusting of plants, but because of severe skin reactions, only rarely in medicine.

RUTIN
Vascular. Greenish yellow powder insoluble in water.
Absorption: From G. I. tract.
Actions and Uses: Said, without good substantiation, to decrease capillary fragility and, therefore, used in cases with purpura, and other evidences of capillary fragility.
Warnings: Not dependable.
Administration: Oral.
Preparations: Tablet, 20 mg.
Dose: 20 mg. 3 times a day.

S

SACCHARIN
Flavor. White powder, soluble in water. About 500 times as sweet as sugar.
Actions and Uses: Sweetening agent. Used as a sugar substitute.
Warnings: Continued use may lead to digestive upset.
Administration: Oral.
Preparations: Tablet, as such and as sodium salt. 15 mg., 30 mg., 60 mg.
Dose: 30 mg.

SAL-ETHYL CARBONATE®, see Carbethyl Salicylate

SALICIM®, see Salicylamide

SALICYLAMIDE—Salicim®, Salrin®
Analgesic. An amide of salicylic acid with the same general pharmacologic and therapeutic properties of the salicylates, which see. Statements of great superiority to other salicylates not confirmed.
Warnings: There is no reason to believe that there is any real superiority between this drug and other members of the group or that it is less toxic or safer in any way. Do not confuse with Salicylanilide, an antifungal agent which is toxic when given by mouth.

SALICYLANILIDE—Ansadol®, Salinidol®
An antifungal agent used topically.
Warnings: Do not confuse with salicylamide, the analgesic agent.

SALICYLATES

Salicylates are a group of drugs, all of which are analgesic in doses which do not impair mental acuity. They are effective against a variety of common pains and aches, as headaches, muscle pains, dysmenorrhea, arthritic pains, etc. Not especially effective against traumatic pains, intestinal pain, migraine headaches and severe pain. They are also effective antipyretics.

As a group, they are among the safest in common use, and that is one of the reasons why widespread use of Aspirin has not led to many accidents. Occasional patients exhibit a hypersensitivity to the salicylates. They are also used in rather large doses to relieve the exquisite pain of rheumatic fever.

The use of sodium bicarbonate together with the salicylates reduces the tendency of large doses to irritate the stomach, and at the same time hastens the rapidity with which it is eliminated from the body.

The common symptoms of overdosage are ringing in the ears, dizziness and nausea. Some of the salicylates have special uses as salicylic acid, phenyl salicylate and methyl salicylate.

Acetylsalicylic acid, Ethyl salicylate, Methyl salicylate, Phenyl salicylate, Salicylamide, Salicylic acid, Sodium salicylate.

SALICYLAZOSULFAPYRIDINE—
Azulfidine®

Sulfonamide. Brownish yellow powder, insoluble in water.

Actions and Uses: Much the same as sulfapyridine. Said to have special value in treatment of ulcerative colitis, but awaits confirmation.

Warnings: Of unproved value on the one hand while, on the other, it shares all of the hazards of sulfapyridine, one of the more toxic sulfonamides. See Sulfonamides.

Administration: Oral.

Preparations: Tablet, 0.5 Gm.

Dose: See Sulfonamides.

SALICYLIC ACID
Salicylate and keratolytic. White powder, slightly soluble in water.

Absorption: From G. I. tract.

Actions and Uses: As other salicylates. Infrequently used internally because of

gastric irritation. Potent keratolytic used in skin preparations to induce peeling of skin or skin lesions.

Warnings: Avoid contact with iron. Do not apply to large areas of the skin.

Administration: Topical.

Preparations: Ointment, cream, collodion and mixed with various other skin preparations.

Dose: Concentration, 3–20%, depending on purpose.

SALINIDOL®, see Salicylanilide

SALOL, see Phenyl Salicylate

SALOPHEN®, see Phenetsal

SALRIN®, see Salicylamide

SALT, see Sodium Chloride

SALVARSAN, see Arsphenamine

SALYRGAN-THEOPHYLLINE®, see Mersalyl and Theophylline

SANDOPTAL®, see Allylbarbital

SANDRIL®, see Reserpine

SANTONIN
Vermifuge. Crystals or white powder, insoluble in water.

Actions and Uses: Formerly used as a vermifuge, but has been replaced by more effective and less toxic modern drugs.

Warnings: May cause convulsions if absorption into the blood stream occurs. Presence of fats in intestinal tract enhances absorption.

SAPONATED CRESOL SOLUTION, see Cresol Solution

SARSAPARILLA
Flavor.

Actions and Uses: Formerly used in rheumatism in which it was ineffective. Now used only as a flavoring agent.

Preparations: Fluidextract and compound sarsaparilla syrup.

SASSAFRAS
Flavor.

Actions and uses: Mildly aromatic flavoring agent. Also used as a carminative.

Preparations: As such and as an oil, Sassafras Oil.

SCARLET RED—Biebrich Scarlet Red
Epithelial stimulant. Dark brown powder, insoluble in water.
Actions and Uses: Used, without good proof, to stimulate epithelization in burns, ulcers, and wounds.
Warnings: Toxic, if applied over very large areas. Not same as scarlet red sulfonate.
Administration: Topical.
Preparations: Ointment.
Dose: Concentration, 1%.

SCILLAREN®, obtained from squill, which see. Also see Digitalis

SCOPOLAMINE—Hyoscine
Sedative, anticholinergic. The hydrobromide, white powder, soluble in water.
Absorption: From G. I. tract.
Actions and Uses: Much the same as atropine, except that it has central sedative rather than a stimulant action; it appears to act well together with barbiturate drugs, and has been used in "twilight sleep" preparations in obstetrics. Also used in Parkinsonism. Decreases flow of saliva. In eye, action is same as atropine, but appears quickly and wears off more rapidly.
Warnings: Toxic symptoms of disorientation, profound depression and delirium may appear. Excessive action may also produce elevation of body temperature, dilated pupils, dry mouth and throat. Danger of glaucoma is present in sensitive patients.
Administration: Subcutaneous, intravenous, oral.
Preparations: Tablet, 0.13-0.6 mg. Solution, 1 cc. ampule containing 1.0 mg.
Dose: Oral, 0.13-1.0 mg. Parenteral, 0.2-1.0 mg.

SECOBARBITAL—Seconal®
One of the rapid-acting barbiturates, which see.

SECONAL®, see Secobarbital

SEIDLITZ POWDERS, see Effer-
vescent Powders, Compound

SELENIUM SULFIDE—Selsun®
Dermatologic. An intensely yellow suspension.
Absorption: Poorly absorbed from skin surfaces but there is the possibility of absorption and toxicity if the material accumulates in folds, crevices or under the nails.
Actions and Uses: Reduces and controls dandruff but does not cure and requires continued use for control. Not effective against ringworm of the scalp.
Warnings: Toxic orally. Wash scalp and skin thoroughly after using. Stains skin.
Administration: Externally as a shampoo.
Preparations: 2.5% suspension.
Dose: 5-10 cc.

SELSUN®, see Selenium Sulfide

SEMIKON®, see Methapyrilene

SEMOXYDINE®, see Methamphetamine

SENECA SNAKEROOT, see
Senega

SENEGA—Seneca Snakeroot
Expectorant and emetic. Pale brown powder with acrid taste.
Actions and Uses: Rarely used in modern medicine. Nauseant expectorant.
Preparations: Fluidextract and syrup.
Dose: Equivalent of 1.0 Gm. of the powdered root.

SENNA
Vegetable laxative. Greenish-yellow powder.
Actions and Uses: Laxative.
Warnings: As with other cathartics, may lead to dependence if used regularly.
Administration: Oral.
Preparations: Fluidextract. Syrup. Compound senna powder, contains senna, sulfur, glycyrrhiza, fennel oil, and sugar.
Dose: Equivalent of 2 Gm. of the powder.

SENOKOT®, see Cassia Pods

SEQUESTRENE®, see Edathamil

SERFIN®, see Reserpine

SEROMYCIN®, see Cycloserine

SERPASIL®, see Reserpine

SERPILOID®, see Reserpine

SESAME OIL
Vehicle. Pale yellow bland oil.
Actions and Uses: Mainly as a vehicle in parenteral preparations of drugs which are oil-soluble.

SIGNEMYCIN®
Proprietary mixture of oleandomycin and tetracycline. Claims have been made that this mixture has synergistic actions that give it special virtues but evidence has been rapidly accumulating that the oleandomycin is relatively ineffective and that any therapeutic effect the mixture may have is largely; if not entirely, due to the tetracycline it contains.

SILICARE®, see Dimethicone

SILICOTE®, see Dimethicone

SILVER
Silver salts have potent antibacterial actions, and this, in general, constitutes their main use. Silver nitrate, for example, has long been used to prevent gonorrheal blindness in the newborn infant.

In general the inorganic silver salts are highly irritant, and in concentrated solution, highly caustic; from this silver nitrate obtains its synonym, lunar caustic. There are a number of organic silver salts which retain antibacterial action, but which are less irritant to tissues, such as the silver protein compounds and silver picrate.

The silver salts are also potent poisons, usually affecting either central nervous system or G.I. tract, causing convulsions, coma, paralysis, depression of vital centers or gastroenteritis.

Silver salts all tend to stain skin and linens badly. Silver salts also attack all protein matter and the potency of silver solutions is quickly reduced by contamination of any sort.

The continued application of silver salts to skin or mucous membranes, or the taking of small doses internally, may lead to a permanent bluish discoloration of the skin, argyria.

SILVER CHLORIDE, COLLOIDAL
—Lunosol®
Antiseptic. Usually in colloidal solution.
Actions and Uses: In dilute solutions for irrigation of urethra and bladder. Infrequently used at present.

SILVER IODIDE, COLLOIDAL
—Neo-Silvol®
Actions and Uses: See silver chloride.

SILVER NITRATE—Lunar Caustic
Antiseptic. White crystals, soluble in water, changing color in the presence of light.
Actions and Uses: A caustic silver material. See Silver.
Warnings: See Silver.
Preparations: Applicator. Stick. Solution, ophthalmic (1%).

SILVER PICRATE—Picragol®
Antiseptic. Yellowish crystals, slightly soluble in water, discolored by sunlight.
Actions and Uses: Much the same as other silver salts. The powder is used in the treatment of vaginitis due to *Monilia albicans* and *Trichomonas vaginalis.* See Silver.
Warnings: The silver may cause argyria, the picrate may cause nephritis.
Administration: Topical.
Preparations: Powder, 1%. Crystals, 100%. Suppository, 0.13 Gm.
Dose: Depends on indication.

SILVER PROTEIN—Algyn®, Argyrol®, Protargin®, Silvol®
Antiseptic.
Actions and Uses: Used mainly for skin and mucous membrane antisepsis. Giving way to more modern antibiotics and chemotherapeutic agents.
Warnings: Store in dark colored bottles away from light. See Silver.

SILVOL®, see Silver Protein

SINAN®, see Mephenesin

SINTRON®, see Acenocoumarin

SITOSTEROLS—Cytellin®
Lipotropic. Enhances excretion of cholesterol and is recommended for its reduction in hypercholesterolemia. Evidence is lacking, however, that it is of practical

value in atherosclerosis or, for that matter, in other conditions with high blood cholesterol levels. Usually administered orally in doses of about 10 Gm. daily, but much larger doses can also be used.

SKELETAL MUSCLE RELAXANTS, see Muscle relaxants, skeletal

SKIODAN®, see Methiodal

SKOPOLATE®, see Methscopolamine

SLAKED LIME, see Calcium Hydroxide

SOAP, HARD—Castile Soap
For discussion of properties of soap see Soap, Medicinal, Soft.

SOAP, MEDICINAL, SOFT—
Green Soap, Soft Soap, Medicinal
Cleansing agent.
Actions and Uses: The standard soaps are used in medicine merely as cleansing agents. They have no important advantages over the soaps sold in commerce except that, perhaps, they are somewhat purer, contain less irritant extraneous material. In general, the soft soap is more efficient as a cleaning agent than the hard soap. Neither form of soap, however, is an effective antiseptic agent; they merely remove soil from the skin. For antiseptic action in soaps, other material such as pHisoHex, must be used. The hard soap is occasionally used for its irritant action in soap solution enema, to help stimulate bowel activity.
Warnings: The excessive use of soaps may dry the skin and lead to dermatoses.
Preparations: Hard soap, Soft soap, Soap liniment, Soap solution.

SODA LIME
Chemical reagent. Used in basal metabolism tests, anesthesia and oxygen therapy units.

SODIUM ACETATE
Diuretic. Colorless crystals soluble in water.
Actions and Uses: Not a particularly de-

pendable diuretic. Rarely used in modern medicine.

SODIUM ACID PHOSPHATE, see Sodium Biphosphate

SODIUM AMINOSALICYLATE, see Para-Aminosalicylic Acid

SODIUM AMYTAL®, see Amobarbital

SODIUM ARSENATE
Dermatologic. White powder, soluble in water.
Actions and Uses: Used in treatment of pemphigus and dermatitis herpetiformis.
Warnings: Has dangers of other arsenicals. See Arsenic.
Administration: Intramuscular.
Preparations: Solution, 1% containing procaine.
Dose: 3 mg., increasing by small increments daily.
Antidote: Dimercaprol.

SODIUM ASCORBATE—
Vitamin C
Vitamin C. White powder, soluble in water. See Ascorbic acid.

SODIUM BENZOATE
Antiseptic and diagnostic. White powder, soluble in water.
Actions and Uses: A mild antiseptic, often used in food preservation because it is practically nontoxic. Used for liver function test.
Warnings: Rarely toxic except in sensitive patients.
Administration: Oral, intravenous.
Preparations: Powder. Ampule, 1.7 Gm. in 20 cc. water.
Dose: Oral, 6 Gm. Intravenous, 1.7 Gm.

SODIUM BICARBONATE
—Baking Soda, Soda
Alkali and digestive. White powder, soluble in water. Bitter taste.
Actions and Uses: Used in hyperacidity of stomach to neutralize acid; to alkalinize urine, especially in connection with sulfonamide therapy, and with certain drugs to decrease gastric irritation. Also used in washes, douches and alkaline

powders of various sorts. Antidote to acid burns and poisoning.

Warnings: Causes "rebound" acidity of stomach. Excessive use may cause alkalosis. Keep in tightly stoppered bottles.

Administration: Oral, intravenous.

Preparations: Powder. Tablet, 0.3 Gm., 0.6 Gm. Solution, sterile. Sippy powders, 1 and 2.

Dose: 2 Gm. or more.

SODIUM BIPHOSPHATE—Acid Sodium Phosphate

Urinary Acidifier. White power, soluble in water. Saline taste.

Actions and Uses: Tends to acidify urine and used whenever acid urine may be needed, as for example, when using methenamine.

Warnings: May cause laxative action in large doses. If drug fails to acidify urine, there is danger of acidosis. Fixed forms together with other medications are not usually recommended. Urine should be frequently examined.

Administration: Oral.

Preparations: Tablet, 0.3 Gm.

Dose: 0.6 Gm., 1–6 times daily, as indicated by urine examination.

SODIUM BORATE—Borax

Antiseptic. White powder, soluble in water.

Actions and Uses: Slightly antiseptic and has detergent action. Used as an external wash.

Warnings: Do not use internally. Highly toxic internally.

Administration: Topical.

Preparations: Bath. Wash. Solution, Dobell's solution.

Dose: Concentration, 1.5%.

SODIUM BROMIDE

Sedative. White powder, soluble in water, salty taste.

Actions and Uses: Has same sedative actions as other bromides, and in common with them, has the dangers of continued bromide use. Drug is fast falling into disuse.

Warnings: Skin rashes are common; high blood levels of bromides may cause serious neurologic and psychologic disturbances. This may occur without easy explanation because many preparations sold over the counter to lay people contain small or large amounts of bromides. Great danger of toxicity in patients on low salt diets.

Administration: Oral.

Preparations: Tablet, 30 mg., 60 mg. Solution, 7.5%. Mixture, such as triple bromide.

Dose: 1 Gm. three times daily.

Antidote: Sodium chloride, mercurial diuretics.

SODIUM CACODYLATE

Hematinic. White powder, soluble in water. Arsenical.

Actions and Uses: Same as other forms of arsenic, in anemia and leukemia. Used relatively infrequently today.

Warnings: Has all dangers of other forms of arsenic. Oral use gives a garlic odor to the breath. See Arsenic.

Administration: Oral, subcutaneous.

Preparations: Powder and solution.

Dose: 60-300 mg.

Antidote: Dimercaprol.

SODIUM CARBONATE— Washing Soda.

Strong alkali.

Actions and Uses: Cleaning agent. Not used in medicine.

SODIUM CHLORIDE—Salt

Electrolyte. White crystals, soluble in water, saline taste.

Actions and Uses: Provides body fluids with highly important electrolyte salt and alkali. Used in electrolyte disturbances of various sorts, heat cramps, Addison's disease of adrenal glands, fluid restoration and in physiologic solutions. Tends to hold water in body to prevent dehydration. Concentrated solutions have irritant action used to sclerose varicose veins.

Warnings: Excessive use may precipitate heart failure symptoms. Large doses in tablet form may cause gastric irritation unless enteric coated.

Administration: Oral, parenteral.

Preparations: Tablet, 0.2 Gm., 0.3 Gm., 0.5 Gm. Physiologic solution, isotonic, Ringer's, lactated Ringer's, Hartmann's. Hypertonic solution, 5%. Also in tablets with dextrose, sodium bicarbonate.
Dose: Oral, 0.6 Gm. as frequently as needed. Parenteral, as indicated by condition. There is a formula which may be used to determine dose needed in hyponatremia based on blood sodium level and body weight.

SODIUM CITRATE
Anticoagulant. White crystals soluble in water, saline taste.
Actions and Uses: Excreted in urine, which it tends to alkalinize. Not frequently used for this purpose at the present time. Also, by reaction with calcium in blood, prevents blood coagulation. This action is used only in the case of blood for preservation and transfusion, and never in the patient himself (as, for example, Dicumarol® is now used). Used for an action on blood vessels in Buerger's disease, for lead poisoning and in infant milk formulas.
Warnings: Overdosage may cause alkalosis, and by an action with calcium, may depress cardiac action and cause tetany.
Administration: Oral, and directly into blood flasks.
Preparations: Tablet, solution and powder.
Dose: Oral, 1 Gm. as frequently as required. Intravenous, 250-1000 cc. of a 2% solution every other day. Anticoagulant, depending on amount of blood treated.
Antidote: Calcium given intravenously.

SODIUM DEHYDROCHOLATE—
Decholin Sodium®
Actions and Uses: See Dehydrocholic Acid.
Administration: Intravenous.
Preparations: Solution, 20%.
Dose: 2 Gm. daily.

SODIUM FLUORIDE
Dental Prophylactic. Used in great dilution, about 1 part per million, in drinking water to prevent dental caries.

SODIUM FOLATE, see Folic Acid

SODIUM FOLVITE®, see Folic Acid

SODIUM GLUTAMATE—
Glutavene®
New drug used principally in encephalopathy due to hepatic disease. It appears to alleviate these symptoms, especially when they are associated with high blood ammonia levels, by facilitating the metabolism of the ammonia. While the extent or the durability of these benefits remains to be established, this drug appears to be a safe one while the gravity of the condition in which it is used is very great. Its trial seems justified, therefore. Dosage is of the order of 30 Gm. per 24 hours by intravenous infusion.

SODIUM GLYCEROPHOSPHATE, see Glycerophosphates

SODIUM GLYCOCHOLATE, see Ox Bile Extract

SODIUM HEPARIN, see Heparin

SODIUM HYDRATE, see Sodium Hydroxide

SODIUM HYDROXIDE—
Caustic Soda, Sodium Hydrate
Caustic alkali.
Actions and Uses: Potent alkali used solely as laboratory reagent.
Warnings: Highly caustic, destroys tissues rapidly. Destroys clothing, especially woolens.
Antidote: Weak acids and water.

SODIUM HYPOCHLORITE
Antiseptic. White powder, soluble in water. Decomposes rapidly, liberating chlorine.
Actions and Uses: Antiseptic usefulness of hypochlorite solutions depends on decomposition and liberation of chlorine. The latter destroys bacteria and to some extent, dissolves dead tissues.
Warnings: Highly irritant, strong bleaching action. Solutions must be freshly prepared, since they deteriorate rapidly on standing. Refrigerate.
Administration: Topical (usually by irrigation).

Preparations: Solution, Labarraque's (2.5%), Dakin's (0.5%).
Dose: Concentrations, 0.5% on tissues. Stronger for antisepsis of instruments.

SODIUM HYPOPHOSPHITE
Tonic. No evidence for such an action.

SODIUM HYPOSULFITE, see
Sodium Thiosulfate

SODIUM INDIGOTINDISULFON-
ATE—Indigo Carmine
Diagnostic. Purple powder, soluble in water.
Actions and Uses: Excreted by the kidneys and used in kidney function tests.
Warnings: Keep away from light.
Administration: Subcutaneous, intramuscular, intravenous.
Preparations: Solution, ampule of 5 cc. of 0.8% strength.
Dose: Subcutaneous, intramuscular, 50-100 mg. (6.25–12.5 cc.). Intravenous, 8–16 mg. (1–2 cc.).

SODIUM IODIDE
Diagnostic. White crystals, soluble in water, salty taste.
Actions and Uses: Source of iodine for treatment of thyroid disease. Salt of choice for intravenous use. Used also because it is opaque to x-ray in urography (retrograde.)
Warnings: Rash may develop in sensitive patients. Overdosage by vein especially if given too rapidly, may precipitate pulmonary edema.
Administration: Oral, intravenous.
Preparations: Solution, 1–3%.
Dose: Oral, 0.3–2.0 Gm. several times daily. Intravenous, 1–2 Gm. in 1% solution. Retrograde urography, 3% solution, amount determined by procedure and simultaneous x-ray.

SODIUM LACTATE
Electrolyte. White powder, soluble in water.
Actions and Uses: Used to supply sodium salt in situations of electrolyte disturbance in which this is needed. Used to treat acidosis. Also used in infant formulas in treating infant acidosis.

Warnings: Overdosage may cause alkalosis.
Administration: Oral, intravenous, subcutaneous.
Preparations: Solution. One-sixth Molar (M/6), isotonic (1.87%) and 11.2%.
Dose: 500 cc. or more as indicated. In infants, as indicated by status of child.

SODIUM LAURYL SULFATE,
see Duponol®, Penetration Cream

SODIUM MENADIOL DIPHOS-
PHATE—Synkayvite®
A derivative of Menadione, which see.

SODIUM MORRHUATE
Sclerotic. Solution containing small amount of preservative.
Actions and Uses: Irritates and scleroses veins; used in the obliteration of varicose veins.
Warnings: Idiosyncrasy should be considered; serious allergic reactions have been reported; always use test dose first. Concentrations over 5% should not be used.
Administration: Intravenous.
Preparations: Ampule, 5 cc. of 5% solution.
Dose: Should not exceed 5 cc. in one day.

SODIUM NITRITE
Vasodilator. White powder, soluble in water.
Actions and Uses: In common with nitrites, dilates smooth muscle. Especially effective in spasm of the coronary arteries. Action is slower to develop and somewhat more prolonged than nitroglycerine.
Warnings: See Nitrites. Overdosage may cause weakness. Continued use may cause methemoglobinemia and blood dyscrasias.
Administration: Oral.
Preparations: Tablet, 30 mg., 60 mg.
Dose: 60 mg.

SODIUM PARA-AMINOSALICY-
LATE, see Para-Aminosalicylic Acid

SODIUM PENTOBARBITAL, see
Pentobarbital

SODIUM PERBORATE
Antiseptic. White powder, salty taste;

decomposes with liberation of oxygen. Used in mouth washes and treatment of oral infections.
Warnings: Should not be used over long period of time as mouth wash.
Administration: Topical.
Preparations: Powder, flavored.
Dose: Concentration, 2%.

SODIUM PHENOBARBITAL, see Phenobarbital

SODIUM PHOSPHATE—
Dibasic Sodium Phosphate
Cathartic. White powder, soluble in water.
Actions and Uses: Mild laxative. Stimulates emptying of gall-bladder.
Warnings: Keep in tightly stoppered container.
Adminstration: Oral.
Preparations: Solution, effervescent granules and powder (dry).
Dose: 4 Gm.

SODIUM PHOSPHATE, ACID, see Sodium Biphosphate

SODIUM PROPIONATE
Antifungal. White powder, soluble in water.
Actions and Uses: As a fungicide in skin infections.
Administration: Topical.
Preparations: Dusting powder, ointment and jelly.
Dose: Concentration, 10%.

SODIUM PSYLLIATE—Sylnasol®
Sclerotic. Sodium salt of fatty acid.
Actions and Uses: Given intravenously it irritates endothelium of veins and causes thrombosis, an effect which may obliterate veins. Used in treatment of varicose veins and hemorrhoids.
Warnings: Serious allergic reactions may develop; use test dose first.
Administration: Intravenous.
Preparations: Vial, containing 5 and 60 cc. of 5% solution.
Dose: 5 cc.

SODIUM RICINOLEATE—Soricin®
Sclerotic. Sodium salt of fatty acid.
Actions and Uses: Irritates endothelial lining of veins and produces thrombosis,

an effect which is used to obliterate varicose veins and hemorrhoids.
Warnings: Serious allergic reactions may occur; always use the test dose first.
Administration: Intravenous.
Preparations: Parenteral solution, 20 cc. vials containing 2% solution.
Dose: 2 to 5 cc. of above solution.

SODIUM SALICYLATE
Analgesic. White powder, soluble in water, salty taste.
Actions and Uses: Same as other salicylates, but somewhat less irritant to stomach than acetylsalicylic acid (Aspirin); used in cases in which large doses are necessary. Combination with sodium bicarbonate reduces irritant action on stomach, but also hastens elimination.
Warnings: Overdosage may cause dizziness, ringing in ears and nausea.
Administration: Oral.
Preparations: Tablet, mixture with sodium bicarbonate and mixture with theobromine which facilitates solution.
Dose: 1 Gm. as frequently as indicated by condition.
Antidote: Sodium bicarbonate.

SODIUM STEARATE
Base. White powder with soapy touch.
Actions and Uses: Used as base for glycerin suppositories. Essentially inert. Not used internally.

SODIUM SULFADIAZINE
Sulfonamide.
Actions and Uses: Soluble and injectable form of sulfadiazine, which see.
Warnings: See Sulfonamides.
Administration: Intravenous.

SODIUM SULFATE—Glauber's Salt
Cathartic. Colorless crystals, soluble in water, salty taste.
Actions and Uses: Cathartic, with no advantages over many others, but in general, more disagreeable than most saline laxatives. Used intravenously as a diuretic.
Warnings: As with other laxatives, there is the danger of dependence developing from continued use.

Administration: Oral, intravenous.
Preparations: Crystals. Solution, 50%.
Dose: Oral, 15–30 Gm. with water. Intravenous, 100-500 cc. of a 4.0% solution.

SODIUM SULFITE
Preservative. Used in preserving foods and solutions and as an ingredient in mouth washes. Now rarely used in treatment of ringworm and pityriasis versicolor.

SODIUM TAUROCHOLATE AND GLYCOCHOLATE, see Ox Bile Extract

SODIUM TETRADECYL SULFATE
—Sotradecol®
Sclerotic. Clear solution, with preservative.
Actions and Uses: Irritates lining of veins and induces thrombosis. Used in obliteration of varicose veins.
Warnings: Extravenous injection may cause severe pain and local necrosis. Test for sensitivity before using.
Administration: Intravenous.
Preparations: Vial, 20 cc. containing 1% or 3%.
Dose: Not more than 6–10 cc. of 3% solution at one time.

SODIUM THIOCYANATE
Hypotensive. See Thiocyanates.

SODIUM THIOSULFATE—
Sodium Hyposulfite, Hypo
Antiseptic and antidote. Colorless crystals, soluble in water.
Actions and Uses: Exerts moderate antifungal action, and used as prophylactic, but useless in treatment. Used in treatment of metal poisoning (mercury and gold), but probably of little value. Also used in cyanide poisoning. Sometimes used in Buerger's disease. Not a particularly valuable drug and of decreasing importance.
Warnings: Excessive use may suppress blood clotting mechanism.
Administration: Topical, oral, intravenous.
Preparations: Solution, 5–10% in 10 cc. ampule. Lotion.

Dose: Oral, intravenous, 1 Gm. Topical, concentration 50%.

SOFT SOAP, MEDICINAL, see Soap, Medicinal, Soft

SOLACTHYL®, see Corticotropin

SOLGANAL®, see Aurothioglucose

SOLUBLE FLUORESCEIN, see Fluorescein Sodium

SOLUBLE GUNCOTTON, see Pyroxylin

SOLUTHRICIN®, see Tyrothricin

SOLU-CORTEF®, see Hydrocortisone

SOLUTION OF BRAIN EXTRACT
—Thromboplastin®
Hemostatic.
Actions and Uses: Accelerates blood clotting and stops bleeding.
Administration: Topical by spray or direct application in sponge.
Preparations: Vial, 20 cc.
Dose: As indicated by condition.

SOLVENTS
Used in the preparation of medications as well as for cleansing purposes, many of the latter are highly toxic.
Acetone, Alcohol, Benzene, Benzine, Carbon tetrachloride, Ether, Isopropyl alcohol, Methyl alcohol (Wood alcohol), Toluene, Toluol, Xylene (Xylol).

SOMATROPIN
The growth or somatotropic hormone of the anterior pituitary.

SOMNOS®, see Chloral hydrate

SORBITAN, see Polysorbate 80

SORICIN®, see Sodium Ricinoleate

SOTRADECOL®, see Sodium Tetradecyl Sulfate

SPACETAB
Proprietary name for a capsule which is so prepared as to confer unusually prolonged action on any drug incorporated in it.

SPANISH FLIES, see Cantharides

SPANSULE
Proprietary name for a capsule which is so prepared as to confer unusually pro-

longed action on any drug incorporated in it.

SPARINE®, see Promazine

SPASMOLYN®, see Mephenesin

SPEARMINT
Flavor.

SPERMACETI
Base for creams.

SPIRIT OF AMMONIA, AROMATIC, see Ammonia

SPIRIT OF PEPPERMINT, see Peppermint

SPIRIT OF TURPENTINE, see Turpentine Oil

SPIRITUS FRUMENTI—Whiskey

SQUILL
Cardiac stimulant. Pale brown powder, bitter taste. Digitalis material.
Actions and Uses: Has essentially same properties of other digitalis materials. It is not well or regularly absorbed and has no advantages over digitalis itself. Used as basis of rat poison for several reasons: is harmless to domestic animals, produces fatal convulsions in rats which have no vomiting mechanism and do not vomit from toxic doses of digitalis materials.
Warnings: Has all dangers of other digitalis materials.
Administration: Oral, parenteral.
Preparations: Squill itself is not used frequently in this country any more. There are, however, purified preparations, such as scillaren, which are used. Fluidextract, sirup, vinegar.
Dose: Equivalent of 0.1 cc. of the fluidextract.

STANGEN®, see Pyrilamine

STANOLONE—Neodrol®
Androgen.
Actions and Uses: The same as testosterone, which see.

STARCH—Amylum
Base.
Actions and Uses: Inert, except as a food. Used as base for ointments and powders.

Preparations: Powder. In addition to the material itself, the glycerite of starch is a pasty, water soluble material which is used as a base for water soluble jellies.

STARCH-DERIVATIVE DUSTING POWDER—Bio-Sorb®
A derivative of starch mixed with magnesium oxide and sodium salts used as a dusting powder for gloves and in other surgical procedures, to avoid the local irritant actions of talcum.

STATICIN®, see Caronamide

STATOMIN®, see Pyrilamine

STEARIC ACID
Base.
Actions and Uses: Used in making ointments and suppositories.

STEARYL ALCOHOL
Emulsifying agent.
Actions and Uses: Used in making hydrophilic ointments and petrolatum.

STECLIN®, see Tetracycline

STERANE®, see Prednisolone

STERISIL®, see Hexetidine

STEROSAN®, see Chlorquinaldol

STIBAMINE GLUCOSIDE — Neostam®
Antiprotozoal and antimony compound. Cream colored powder soluble in water.
Actions and Uses: Said to be less toxic than other organic antimony materials used for the same purpose. See Antimony.
Warnings: In common with other antimony compounds, may cause serious reactions: vomiting, diarrhea, anaphylactoid reactions, urticaria, collapse. Contraindicated in patients with pneumonia, jaundice, nephritis or ascites. Use only fresh solutions; not after one hour.
Administration: Intravenous.
Preparations: Vial, 0.1 and 0.5 Gm. to be dissolved just before using.
Dose: 0.1 Gm. per 45 Kg. (100 lbs.) body weight.
Antidote: Probably dimercaprol although not yet established.

STIBOPHEN—Fuadin®
Antimony chemotherapeutic. White pow-

der, soluble in water. Deteriorates in light.
Actions and Uses: For treatment of such tropical diseases as schistosomiasis, leishmaniasis and granuloma inguanale.
Warnings: May cause headache. Do not expose solutions to light. Discard solutions if not clear.
Administration: Intramuscular.
Preparations: Ampule, 300 mg. in 5 cc.
Dose: 120 mg. the first day, increasing daily until about a total of 40 cc. (2.5 Gm.) has been given. Other schedules are also used.
Antidote: Probably dimercaprol, although not yet established.

STIGMONENE®, see Benzpyrinium

STILBAMIDINE
Anticarcinogenic. Highly toxic agent used almost exclusively in treatment of multiple myeloma. May give relief from the pain but does not cure, and it is questionable whether it prolongs life.

STILBESTROL, see Diethylstilbestrol

STILPHOSTROL®, see Diethylstilbestrol

STOMACH, POWDERED
Hematinic. Dry powdered defatted wall of hog stomach. Standardized in U.S.P. Units.
Actions and Uses: Treatment of pernicious anemia. This preparation has largely given way to relatively more concentrated forms of replacement therapy.
Preparations: Capsule, although this preparation has largely given way to relatively more concentrated forms of replacement therapy.

STORAX
Parasiticide. Gray-brown, semi-liquid, softened by heat, insoluble in water.
Actions and Uses: Resembles balsam of Peru. Used to treat scabies and other skin parasites.
Administration: Topical.
Preparations: Ointment.
Dose: Concentration, 25% (1 Gm. per dose).

STOVARSOL®, see Acetarsone

STRAMONIUM—Jamestown Weed, Jimson Weed
Antiasthmatic. Powdered dried leaves.
Actions and Uses: Used in many forms for the relief of asthmatic attacks, internally, by smoking or inhaling vapors and fumes.
Warnings: Not especially reliable, and now less commonly used for this reason.
Administration: Oral, inhalation.
Preparations: Capsule, extract, fluidextract, tincture and also sold over the counter to patients in cigarettes and leaves to burn much like incense.
Dose: 75 mg. of the leaf or its equivalent.

STREPTOMYCIN—Strycin®
Antibiotic. White powder, soluble in water.
Actions and Uses: All remarks apply equally well to the derivative, dihydrostreptomycin, which has also the advantage of reduced toxicity. Streptomycin is one of the effective antibiotics. It is not as potent as penicillin in some diseases, in which case, the latter is to be preferred. But, on the other hand, it is effective in diseases not at all helped by penicillin, such as many urinary tract infections, tuberculosis, leprosy, Friedländer's pneumonia, hemophilus influenzae, meningitis, etc. Its disadvantages compared with penicillin, lie in its toxicity and development of bacterial tolerance with amazing speed.
Warnings: Drug of considerable toxicity; overdosage or sensitivity may cause dizziness, complete loss of sense of balance, renal damage, deafness. In addition, bacteria soon develop tolerance (tolerant strains are bred out), and drug becomes valueless. Therefore, on the one hand, treatment must be intensive and effective to prevent development of tolerance, while on the other hand, large doses may cause toxic symptoms. Toxicity is especially likely to develop in elderly patients and those with defective kidney function.
Administration: Intramuscular, intrathecal.

133

SUCCINYLCHOLINE

Preparations: Ampule, containing 1 Gm. of the base. (Also dihydrostreptomycin.)
Dose: 2–4 Gm. daily.

STRONTIUM LACTATE—Strontolac®
Evidence has been presented that strontium may be an effective adjuvant to calcium therapy in cases of osteoporosis in which calcium alone is ineffective. Usually the strontium is given together with the standard forms of treatment for the osteoporosis, calcium, vitamin D, estrogens, androgens, high protein diet, etc.
Preparations: Capsule, 0.7 Gm.
Dose: About 2.0 Gm. 3 times a day.

STRONTIUM SALTS
Actions and Uses: These are bromides and salicylates with no particular advantages over the more common bromides and salicylates; rarely used today.

STRONTOLAC®, See Strontium Lactate

STROPHANTHIN—Strophanthin K
Cardiac stimulant. White powder, soluble in water.
Absorption: Poorly absorbed from G. I.
Actions and Uses: Typical digitalis material, poorly absorbed from G. I. tract. Used only by parenteral injection. Far more commonly used in Europe than in this country. Develops effects rather rapidly after injection, and these effects are quickly dissipated.
Warnings: As for all other digitalis materials.
Administration: Intravenous.
Dose: 0.5 mg.

STROPHANTHIN G, see Ouabain

STROPHANTHIN K, see Strophanthin

STRYCHNINE
Convulsant. White powder. Salts (nitrate, phosphate, sulfate) are soluble; all intensely bitter.
Actions and Uses: Long been used as a stimulant and tonic. It stimulates the spinal reflex, but there is no evidence that it has any therapeutic value; disappearing from modern medicine. Still used as a rat and mouse poison.
Warnings: Highly toxic agent causing tetanic convulsions with opisthotonus. There are some medications which contain small amounts not toxic to adults (such as cathartic pills which contain strychnine), which may be fatal if taken in sufficient number by infants.
Dose: Safe dose, 1–2 mg. for an adult.
Antidote: Ether, alcohol, barbiturates.

STRYCIN®, see Streptomycin

STYRONATE RESINS—Katonium®
Exchange resin. Light brown powder, insoluble in water. Vanilla flavor, slight aromatic odor.
Absorption: Not absorbed from G.I. tract.
Actions and Uses: Binds and removes cations, particularly sodium, from G.I. tract. Resulting decrease of sodium level in body fluids promotes diuresis and causes edema to subside. Contains ammonium and potassium resins. In return for the cations which become linked with it, it releases potassium and ammonium ions. Some of the latter combine with chloride ions to form ammonium chloride, the diuretic effect of which reinforces the action of the resin.
Warnings: Administered in cold beverages to improve palatability. Make a paste of the powder and then add solution to about 6 ounces in drinking glass. Should be well stirred and administered immediately.
Administration: Oral.
Preparations: Powder, packets of 15 Gm.
Dose: 15 Gm. 2-3 times daily.

SUAVITIL®, see Benactyzine

SUCARYL®, see Cyclamate

SUCCINYLCHOLINE—Anectine®, Quelicin®, Sucostrin®
Muscle relaxant. The chloride, a white slightly bitter powder, soluble in water.
Actions and Uses: Produces muscle relaxation much like that of the curariform drugs but by a different mechanism. Used in anesthesia and electro-shock therapy. Action is relatively brief.

Warnings: Because of respiratory depression must not be used unless adequate provision is made for artificial respiration. Neostigmine and edrophobium must not be used as antagonists for they may intensify its action. Use with caution in patients with liver disease, anemia and malnutrition.
Administration: Intravenous by slow drip or single injection.
Preparations: Vials, 10 cc., containing 20 mg. per cc.
Dose: 20 mg.

SUCCINYLSULFATHIAZOLE—
Sulfasuxidine®
Chemotherapeutic.
Actions and Uses: Poorly absorbed sulfonamide, used in intestinal antisepsis, as a preliminary to surgery and against bacillary infections. See Sulfonamides.
Warnings: Sometimes well absorbed, in which case the same dangers as with other sulfonamides exist. Hypersensitivity may be present with even these poorly absorbed sulfonamides. See Sulfonamides.
Administration: Oral.
Preparations: Tablet, 0.3 Gm., 0.5 Gm.
Dose: 2.0 Gm. daily.

SUCOSTRIN®, see Succinylcholine

SUCROSE—Cane Sugar
Flavor. Colorless crystals with sweet taste. Soluble in water.
Actions and Uses: Flavoring agent, in sirups, elixirs, etc. Occasionally used as a diuretic, which action it exerts by preventing reabsorption of water in the kidney. Used in concentrated solution to reduce elevated intracranial pressure or intraocular pressure (glaucoma), which it does by much the same action.
Warnings: There is evidence that the repeated intravenous use of this material may cause permanent kidney damage. Discard unclear solutions.
Administration: Oral, intravenous.
Preparations: Crystals. Syrup. Solution.
Dose: Intravenous, 200–300 cc. of 50% solution.

SUGAR OF LEAD, see Lead
Acetate

SULAMYD®, see Sulfacetamide

SULESTREX®, see Estrone

SULESTREX PIPERAZINE®, see Piperazine Estrone Sulfate

SULFACETAMIDE—Sulamyd®
Chemotherapeutic. White powder, which for a sulfonamide is very soluble in water.
Available as such and as sodium salt.
Actions and Uses: Because of easy solubility recommended for urinary tract infections.
Warnings: There is no evidence, that but for its solubility it has any advantage over other less soluble sulfonamides or that it carries less danger from other reactions. See Sulfonamides.

SULFADIAZINE
Chemotherapeutic. White powder, insoluble; sodium salt very soluble.
Actions and Uses: Typical actions of the well-absorbed sulfonamides. If precautions are taken to insure complete solution in urine, it is the sulfonamide of choice for systemic infections. High concentrations attained in cerebrospinal fluid after oral administration, making it especially useful in meningitis. See Sulfonamides.
Warnings: Highly insoluble, alkalinize urine and force fluids; watch for hypersensitivity and blood dyscrasias. See Sulfonamides.
Administration: Oral and parenteral.
Preparations: Tablets, 0.5 Gm. Vials of sodium salt.
Dose: 2.0–4.0 Gm. daily in divided doses.

SULFA DRUGS, see Sulfonamides

SULFAETHYLTHIADIAZOLE—
Sul-Spansion®
Sulfonamide. Available in a sustained-release suspension and recommended for urinary tract infections. Special virtues are yet to be demonstrated.

SULFAGUANIDINE
Chemotherapeutic.
Absorption: Poorly absorbed sulfonamide.
Actions and Uses: Used for therapy of infections of G. I. tract. See Sulfonamides.
Warnings: See Sulfonamides.

SULFAMERAZINE
Chemotherapeutic.
Actions and Uses: Same as sulfadiazine although it has been stated that it is somewhat more slowly eliminated and dosage need not be as frequent. See Sulfonamides.
Warnings: See Sulfonamides.

SULFAMETHAZINE
Chemotherapeutic.
Sulfonamide drug with properties similar to sulfamerazine, which see. See Sulfonamides.

SULFAMETHIZOLE—
Thiosulfil®
Chemotherapeutic.
A new highly soluble sulfonamide drug recommended for the treatment of infections of the urinary tract. It may be presumed that it has the advantages and disadvantages of the other very soluble sulfonamides. See Sulfonamides.

SULFANILAMIDE
Chemotherapeutic.
Actions and Uses: The mother substance; rarely used because it is less effective than most of the other sulfonamides. See Sulfonamides.
Warnings: See Sulfonamides.

SULFAPYRAZINE
Chemotherapeutic.
Actions and Uses: Much the same as sulfadiazine although it is stated that elimination is slow and dosage is needed less frequently. See Sulfonamides.
Warnings: See Sulfonamides.

SULFAPYRIDINE
Chemotherapeutic.
Actions and Uses: An early sulfonamide, now rarely used because of relatively high toxicity. See Sulfonamides.
Warnings: See Sulfonamides.

SULFASUXIDINE®, see Succinyl-sulfathiazole

SULFATHALIDINE®, see Phthal-ylsulfathiazole

SULFATHIAZOLE
Chemotherapeutic.
Actions and Uses: Much the same as sulfadiazine although it is stated that it

is somewhat more toxic. It is said to be more effective than other sulfonamides in staphylococcic infections. Little used at present. See Sulfonamides.
Warnings: See Sulfonamides.

SULFA-TRIAZINE®, see Trisulfa-pyrimidines

SULFID®, see Phenylazodiamino-pyridine

SULFISOMIDINE—Elkosin®
Chemotherapeutic.
Actions and Uses: Same as for other Sulfonamides, which see.

SULFISOXAZOLE—Gantrisin®
Chemotherapeutic and urinary antiseptic.
Highly soluble sulfonamide.
Actions and Uses: Used for urinary tract infections, especially in elderly patients and infants. See Sulfonamides.
Warnings: See Sulfonamides.

SULFOBROMOPHTHALEIN
—Bromsulphalein®
Diagnostic. White powder, soluble in water, bitter taste.
Actions and Uses: For liver function test.
Administration: Intravenous.
Preparations: Ampule, 3 cc. size, containing 50 mg. per cc.
Dose: 5 mg. (0.1 cc.) per Kg. of body weight.

SULFONAMIDES
These are now a large list of closely related chemotherapeutic compounds selected from perhaps 6000 drugs which were synthesized and screened. Those rejected were either ineffective or toxic. Of the sulfa drugs which remain in use today, most are more or less equally effective in the diseases for which they are used. The choice is determined by individual idiosyncrasy, absorption, rate of elimination, solubility in urine and bone marrow sensitivity.
The sulfonamides may be divided into three groups: (1) poorly absorbed drugs used for intestinal diseases; (2) highly soluble drugs for urinary tract infections, infants and elderly patients; (3) generally chemotherapeutic agents.
Kidney damage can be largely avoided

by attention to the complete solution of drug in the urine. Keeping urine alkaline is a device for this purpose, as is also the mixture of the sulfonamides. In the case of the poorly absorbed sulfonamides this danger does not exist.

In all cases the danger of bone marrow depression is a real one and must be constantly considered and watched by regular red and white cell counts.

In many instances penicillin is preferred only because it does not present these hazards. At present the sulfa drugs are outstanding in treatment of meningococcus meningitis and some urinary tract infections.

The sulfonamides are not generally recommended for topical application because they not only delay healing but also because there is good evidence that they are much more effective when taken systemically.

Nearly all sulfa drugs come in 0.5 Gm. tablets. Sodium salts are available for parenteral injections.

Sulfonamides: Phenazothiadiazine, Phthalylsulfathiazole, Para-nitrosulfathiazole, Salicylazosulfapyridine, Succinylsulfathiazole, Sulfacetamide, Sulfadiazine, Sulfaethylthiadiazole, Sulfamethazine, Sulfamethylthiadiazole, Sulfisomidine, Sulfisoxazole.

Sulfonamide mixtures: Sulfadiazine and Sulfamerazine, Trisulfapyrimidines, (Sulfadiazine, Sulfamerazine, Sulfamethazine).

SULFONES
A group of drugs, related to the sulfonamides, which are effective in leprosy and also sometimes used in tuberculosis. Diaminodiphenylsulfone, Glucosulfone, Sulfoxone, Thiazolsulfone.

SULFOXONE—Diasone®
Sulfone. Used principally in the treatment of leprosy. Toxic effects are common. Usual dosage is from 0.3 to 0.6 Gm. daily.

SULFUR DIOXIDE
Gas.
Actions and Uses: Rarely used. Used externally in solution as a parasiticide.

Used internally in the treatment of pyrosis.

SULFUR, PRECIPITATED
Parasiticide and antifungal. Yellow powder, insoluble in water.
Actions and Uses: Externally in many skin preparations for its action against parasites, fungi and other skin diseases. Used internally, it is a mild cathartic and despite its traditional remedial values is unimportant in internal medicine.
Warnings: Excessive use on the skin may cause dermatitis.
Administration: Topical, oral.
Preparations: Lotion, ointment, mixture of various types, sublimed sulfur, washed sulfur, all having the same values.
Dose: Oral, 4 Gm. Topical, concentrations 6–30%.

SUL-SPANSION®, see Sulfaethylthiadiazole

SUMYCIN®, see Tetracycline Phosphate Complex

SUPERINONE—Alevaire®
Liquifier. Detergent, available in sterile solution. Used mainly to liquify pulmonary secretions. Administered only by nebulizer, both intermittently and continuously.

SURAMIN—Naphuride®
Antiprotozoal. White powder with bitter taste; the sodium salt, soluble in water. Deteriorates in presence of light.
Actions and Uses: Treatment of and prophylaxis of African trypanosomiasis. Also used in the treatment of pemphigus.
Warnings: Kidney irritant. May also damage the adrenals. Examine blood and urine for signs of toxicity. Use only freshly prepared solutions.
Administration: Intravenous.
Preparations: Ampule, containing 1 Gm. to be dissolved before using.
Dose: 1 Gm. weekly.

SURFACAINE®, see Cyclomethycaine

SURGICAL PITUITRIN, see Pituitary, Posterior

SURGI-CEN®, see Hexachlorphene

SURITAL®, see Thiamylal

SWEET ALMOND OIL, see Almond Oil, Expressed

SWEET BIRCH OIL, see Methyl Salicylate

SYLNASOL®, see Sodium Psylliate

SYNANDROL®, see Testosterone

SYNATAN®, see Tanphetamine

SYMPATHOMIMETICS, see Adrenergics

SYNCELOSE®, see Methylcellulose

SYNCURINE®, see Decamethonium

SYNDROX®, see Methamphetamine

SYNESTROL®, see Dienestrol

SYNGESTERONE®, see Progesterone

SYNKAYVITE®, see Sodium Menadiol Diphosphate

SYNTHETIC OLEOVITAMIN D —Viosterol, Drisdol®
Vitamin. Solution in sesame oil, expressed in U.S.P. Units.
Actions and Uses: Same as other forms of vitamin D. For prevention and treatment of ricketts. Use in arthritis and other diseases not clearly a result of vitamin deficiency is dubious. Adult requirements under ordinary circumstances are very small since their bones are already fully formed, but in special instances, such as pregnancy and diseases with poor absorption, or calcium loss, more than the normal amount of the vitamin may be required. It has no general tonic action.
Warnings: There is danger from large overdosage. Manufacturer must indicate whether preparation contains calciferol or other form of vitamin D.
Administration: Oral.
Preparations: Too numerous to describe: capsules, tablets, oily solutions, mixtures, etc.
Dose: Varies with condition. From 500 Units to 10,000 Units daily, with exceptional instances requiring larger doses.

SYNTHYROID SODIUM®, see Levothyroxine Sodium

SYNTOPHYLATE®, see Theophylline Sodium Glycinate

SYNTROPAN®, see Amprotropine

T

TACE®, see Chlorotrianisene

TAGATHEN®, see Chlorothen

TALBUTAL—Lotusate®
One of the rapid-acting barbiturate drugs, which see. Available in 30, 50 and 120 mg. capsules. The first two being sedative doses, the last the average hypnotic dose.

TALC—Talcum
Protective. Fine white or grayish powder. Insoluble in water.
Actions and Uses: Protective and absorbent in skin irritations and eruptions.
Warnings: May cause severe tissue reactions in wounds and body cavities, and is no longer used, therefore, for dusting surgical gloves.
Administration: Topical.
Preparations: Powder.

TALCUM, see Talc

TANNIC ACID—Gallotannic Acid
Astringent and antidote. Soluble, brown powder.
Actions and Uses: Astringent on the skin. Formerly used in treatment of burns, but has been discontinued because of evidence of liver damage from extensive use. Antidote in metal and alkaloid poisoning. Also a hemostatic to control bleeding and orally to control diarrhea.
Warnings: Solutions are unstable. Application over large denuded surfaces may cause liver damage. Avoid contact with metals.
Administration: Topical, oral.
Preparations: Solution, glycerite and suppository.
Dose: Oral, 0.2–0.6 Gm. in solution. Topical, concentrations 2–50%.

TANPHETAMINE—Synatan®
Adrenergic. Complex of Dextroamphetamine, which see, with same but prolonged actions.

TAPAZOLE®, see Metimazole

TAR, COAL, see Coal Tar

TAR, JUNIPER, see Juniper Tar

TARTAR EMETIC, see Antimony Potassium Tartrate

TARTARIC ACID
Pharmaceutic. Used mainly in pharmaceutical preparations as source of acid.
Warnings: May injure the kidneys.

TAUROCHOLIC AND GLYCO-CHOLIC ACIDS, see Ox Bile Extract

TEA, see Tetraethylammonium

TELAPAQUE®, see Iopanoic Acid

TELDRIN®, see Chlorpheniramine

TEM, see Triethylene Melamine

TENSILON®, see Edrophonium

TERFONYL®, see Trisulfapyrimidines

TERIDAX®, see Iophenoxic Acid

TERPIN HYDRATE
Expectorant. Crystals or white powder, slightly soluble in water.
Actions and Uses: Used largely as an expectorant.
Warnings: May irritate stomach.
Administration: Oral.
Preparations: Elixir of terpin hydrate, with and without codeine.
Dose: 0.25 Gm. or 4 cc. of elixir.

TERRAMYCIN®, see Oxytetracycline

TESTANDRONE®, see Testosterone

TESTOBASE®, see Testosterone

TESTOSTEROID®, see Testosterone

TESTOSTERONE—Androlin®, Andronaq®, Andronate®, Andrusol®, Malestrone®, Masenate®, Mertestate®, Neo-Hombreol®, Oreton®, Perandren®, Synandrol®, Testandrone®, Testobase®, Testosteroid®, Testrone®, Testryl®

Androgen. As such, the cyclopropionate and the propionate.
Insoluble in water.
Actions and Uses: Replaces deficient male hormone in cases of insufficiency or male menopause, natural or surgical. In the female may be used in cases of excessive menstrual bleeding and carcinoma of the breast.
Warnings: In young males, may induce premature sexual stimulation. In females may induce virilism. In adult males may induce priapism.
Administration: Intramuscular, implantation (rarely used at present).
Preparations: Oil solution, water suspension.
Dose: Intramuscular, 25 mg., or more or less depending on particular indication. Implantation, 0.3 Gm. of testosterone every few months.

TESTOSTERONE ENANTHATE—Delatestryl®
Androgen. Said to have especially prolonged androgenic action. Real advantages over forms of testosterone already available remain to be established. Available in oily solution for intramuscular injection.

TESTRONE®, see Testosterone

TESTRYL®, see Testosterone

TETRABON®, see Tetracycline

TETRACAINE—Pontocaine®
Surface anesthetic. The hydrochloride, white powder, soluble in water. Bitter taste.
Actions and Uses: Local anesthetic for surface anesthesia. Absorbed from mucous membranes and denuded surfaces. Also for spinal anesthesia. Does not dilate pupil, hence, often used in ophthamology for anesthesia.
Warnings: More potent than cocaine; dose must be adjusted accordingly. Rapidly absorbed from mucous membranes, may cause central effects from extensive topical application.
Administration: Topical, intrathecal.
Preparations: Solution, with dropper for

ophthalmic use, 1%. Ointment, 1%. Sterile solution, 1%.
Dose: For spinal anesthesia, 20–40 mg.
Antidote: Epinephrine, barbiturates, artificial respiration.

TETRACHLORETHYLENE
Vermifuge. Colorless liquid with characteristic odor. Insoluble in water. Readily soluble in presence of fat.
Actions and Uses: For hookworm infestations.
Warnings: Highly toxic drug. Should not be given if fats, oils or alcohol are taken at the same time. Should not be used in alcoholics. May cause liver damage.
Administration: Oral.
Preparations: Capsule, 0.2, 1.0, 2.5 cc.
Dose: 3 cc. followed by saline cathartic.

TETRACYCLINE — Achromycin®, Panmycin®, Polycycline®, Steclin®, Tetrabon®, Tetracyn®
A derivative of chlortetracycline and differing very little in antibiotic activity or therapeutic utility from oxytetracycline and chlortetracycline. Dosage and schedule of treatment also the same. There is evidence that tetracycline may be absorbed higher in the gastrointestinal tract as well as more completely than other broad-spectrum antibiotics, so that it causes fewer disturbances by an action on the lower bowel. This is probably the greatest advantage of this drug over other similar antibiotics. There may also be some instances in which a patient cannot tolerate either oxytetracycline or chlortetracycline but may do well on the tetracycline. Administered orally and parenterally.

TETRACYCLINE PHOSPHATE BUFFERED—Achromycin V®, Panmycin Phosphate®, Tetracyn V®
The precise value of the phosphate buffering of tetracycline is not clear and, until this is clarified, it should be assumed to differ little from tetracycline as such.

TETRACYCLINE PHOSPHATE COMPLEX—Sumycin®, Tetrex®
Antibiotic. The advantages of the phosphate complex over the regular tetracyline are not established and, until then, it should be assumed that they are much the same.

TETRACYN®, see Tetracycline

TETRACYN V®, see Tetracycline Phosphate Buffered

TETRAETHYLAMMONIUM—TEA, Etamon®
Anticholinergic and adrenolytic.
White powder, the chloride, soluble in water.
Actions and Uses: Depresses both sympathetic and parasympathetic impulses, causing peripheral vasodilatation; used in vasospastic disease.
Warnings: May cause palpitations, hypotension, shock.
Administration: Intravenous, intramuscular.
Preparations: Vials, 20 cc. of 1:1000 solution.
Dose: 10–15 mg. per Kg. body weight.

TETRAHYDROZOLIDINE— Tyzine®
Nasal decongestant belonging to the adrenergic group but said to exert systemic effects rarely and to exert prolonged local action.

TETREX®, see Tetracycline Phosphate Complex

THEELIN®, see Estrone

THEELOL®, see Estriol

THELESTRIN®, see Estrone

THENFADIL®, see Thenyldiamine

THENYLDIAMINE—Thenfadil®
Antihistamine. Dosage of the order of 15 to 100 mg.

THENYLENE®, see Methapyrilene

THEOBROMA OIL—Cacao Butter, Cocoa Butter
Pharmaceutic. Base for suppositories and sometimes in ointments.

THEOBROMINE AND SODIUM ACETATE—Thesodate®
A theobromine salt claimed to be better tolerated by the G.I. tract than other Xanthine derivatives. There is consider-

able difference of opinion over this blanket claim, many feeling that it has no special advantages. See Theobromine and Sodium salicylate.

THEOBROMINE AND SODIUM SALICYLATE—Diuretin®
Xanthine and diuretic. Calcium salicylate, sodium acetate, sodium salicylate forms. White powder with bitter taste, whose solubility is enhanced by addition of above mentioned salts.

Actions and Uses: In common with other xanthines, has diuretic action, central stimulant action and some tendency to elevate blood pressure. In theobromine preparations the diuretic action is well developed, the others not as much as in the case of caffeine. Even so, it is not as potent or dependable as the mercurial diuretics.

Warnings: Not a dependable diuretic. Large doses often cause gastric distress.
Administration: Oral.
Preparations: Tablet, of the above salts.
Dose: 1 Gm. 3 times daily.

THEOGLYCINATE®, see Theophylline-Sodium Glycinate

THEOPHYLLINE AND SODIUM ACETATE
Xanthine. See Aminophylline.

THEOPHYLLINE ETHYLENE-DIAMINE, see Aminophylline

THEOPHYLLINE-METHYLGLU-CAMINE—Glucophylline®
Xanthine. See Aminophylline.

THEOPHYLLINE-SODIUM GLY-CINATE—Cinaphyl®, Dorsaphyllin®, Glynazan®, Glytheonate®, Syntophylate®, Theoglycinate®
Xanthine. See Aminophylline.

THEOSODATE®, see Theobromine Sodium Acetate

THEPHORIN®, see Phenindamine

THIAMIN—Vitamin B₁
Vitamin. Hydrochloride, white powder, characteristic odor. Soluble in water.
Absorption: Well absorped from G. I. tract.

Actions and Uses: In diseases due to vitamin deficiency, such as beri beri, and other less definitive forms. In other cases of vitamin deficiencies, since there are rarely pure vitamin deficiencies. Used in prevention of vitamin deficiency. It seems to be of value in various forms of neuritis, in which, for dietary or metabolic reasons, there is a relative deficiency of vitamin B₁.

Warnings: Allergic sensitivity may develop, especially after parenteral use. Intramuscular injections are usually painful.
Administration: Oral, intramuscular, intravenous.
Preparations: Tablet, capsule, 3, 5, 10, 25, 50, 100 mg. Sterile solution.
Dose: Varies widely depending on indications.

THIAMYLAL—Surital®
One of the very rapid acting barbiturates, which see.

THIAZOLSULFONE—Promizole®
Sulfone. Used in the treatment of leprosy. A new drug with special hazards, including thyroid enlargement and, after prolonged treatment in young people, abnormal development of secondary sex characteristics. Dosage ranges around 4 to 6 Gm. daily by mouth.

THIMECIL®, see Methylthiouracil

THIMEROSAL—Merthiolate®
Mercurial antiseptic.
Actions and Uses: In common with other organic mercurial antiseptics, it is less irritant and corrosive than mercuric salts, but cannot be depended on to produce complete local antisepsis. It is commonly used as household antiseptic agent.
Warnings: Not to be taken internally.
Administration: Topical.
Preparations: Solution, tincture, vaginal tampons and suppository.
Dose: Concentration, 1:1000 to 1:30,000.
Antidote: Dimercaprol.

THIO-BISMOL®, see Bismuth Sodium Thioglycollate

THIOCYANATES
These drugs were used for reduction of

blood pressure in patients with essential hypertension. There are many dangers and the blood levels of thiocyanate must be carefully watched if serious reactions are to be avoided. Results have not been satisfactory and, as a result, the drugs have been used progressively less with the passage of time.

THIOMERIN®, see Mercaptomerin

THIOPENTAL—Pentothal®
Fixed anesthetic and barbiturate. Yellowish powder, soluble in water. Disagreeable odor.

Actions and Uses: This is one of the rapidly acting barbiturates which is used as a general anesthetic, or a preanesthetic, because it induces anesthesia, by intravenous injection, pleasantly, and its effects wear off rapidly after the operation is concluded. Because of its rapid action, however, the material has to be given continuously during operation. It does not always provide the degree of muscular relaxation needed for surgery, and in such instances some other agents must also be used.

Warnings: Solutions deteriorate very rapidly. Inject very slowly.
Administration: Intravenous.
Preparations: Ampule, containing 0.5, 1.0, 5.0 Gm. to be dissolved before using.
Dose: To be determined by the needs of operator by the anesthetist.
Antidote: Picrotoxin or, if shock develops, parenteral fluids.

THIOSULFIL®, see Sulfamethizole
THIOURACIL DERIVATIVES
These represent a group of drugs related to thiouracil which depress activity of thyroid gland and are used in treatment of hyperthyroidism. Propylthiouracil and some of the others are less toxic than the original thiouracil and the latter has, therefore, been largely discarded. The use of these drugs may lead to the enlargement of the thyroid gland. In most instances these drugs are used preliminary to surgery but there are some cases of hyperthyroidism which can be treated with these drugs alone. In some sensitive

patients danger of agranulocytosis exists, although it has been considerably reduced by the introduction of newer derivatives of thiouracil. In cases resistant to one preparation there is the possibility of good response to another.
Methimazole, Methylthiouracil, Propylthiouracil, Thiouracil, Iodo-thiouracil.

THIXOKON®, see Acetrizoate
THONZYLAMINE—Neohetramine®
One of the large series of antihistamine drugs, which see.

THORAZINE®, see Chlorpromazine
THREE CHLORIDES SOLUTION, see Ringer's Solution
THROMBIN
Hemostatic. White powder.
Actions and Uses: To control bleeding during operation.
Warnings: Not to be injected. Examine label for expiration date.
Administration: Topical in solution or as powder.
Preparations: Ampule, containing 5000 Iowa units to be dissolved in 5 cc. sterile saline just before using.
Dose: Concentration, 100-2000 units per cc.

THRCMBOPLASTIN®, see Solution of Brain Extract
THYLOGEN®, see Pyrilamine
THYLOSE®
Sodium carboxy-methylcellulose. See methylcellulose.
THYME
Counterirritant and diaphoretic. The leaf or the oil, with characteristic taste and odor.
Actions and Uses: Counterirritant, usually the oil in a liniment. As a diaphoretic and in nostrums. Not frequently used in modern medicine.
Administration: Oral.
Preparations: Fluidextract, sirup, oil.
Dose: Equivalent of 4.0 Gm. of the leaf.
THYMOL
Vermifuge and antiseptic. Crystals with characteristic odor and taste. Slightly soluble in water.

Actions and Uses: Antiseptic and anthelmintic against tapeworms.
Warnings: Highly toxic, especially together with fats, oils and alcohol. Use cautiously in alcoholic patients.
Administration: Oral.
Preparations: Crystals in capsule.
Dose: 2 Gm. divided into 3 doses.

THYMOL IODIDE—Aristol®
Dusting powder. Reddish powder with characteristic odor.
Actions and Uses: Antiseptic dusting powder.
Warnings: Deteriorates in direct light. Store in amber bottles. Not for internal use. There is danger of allergic reaction in sensitive patients. See Iodine.

THYROID—Dessicated Thyroid Extract
Hormone. Yellowish powder from glands of cattle.
Absorption: Well absorbed from G. I. tract.
Actions and Uses: Exerts same effects as action of thyroid gland; used in disease of thyroid insufficiency, such as cretinism, myxedema and less pronounced thyroid insufficiencies. Use in treatment of obesity requires constant attention to prevent serious reactions.
Warnings: Overdosage causes hyperthyroidism.
Administration: Oral.
Preparations: Tablet, 15, 30, 60 mg.
Dose: As indicated by conditions. Average 60 mg. daily.

THYROTROPIN—Thytropar®
Hormone. Stimulates thyroid activity; used in special thyroid disturbances. Available as a lyophilized powder to be made up before use.

THYTROPAR®, see Thyrotropin

THYROXIN
A purified and potent extract of thyroid gland which represents one of the precursors of the actual thyroid hormone. Rarely used in clinical medicine.

TISIN®, see Isoniazid

TOCLASE®, see Carbetapentane

TOLANATE®, see Inositol Hexanitrate
TOLANSIN®, see Mephenesin
TOLAZOLINE—Priscoline®
Vasodilator and adrenolytic. Soluble white powder.
Absorption: Absorbed from G. I. tract.
Actions and Uses: By blocking sympathetic ganglia, prevents and relieves constriction of peripheral vessels. Used in vasoconstriction due to thrombosis, embolism, and in vasospastic diseases such as Raynaud's disease.
Warnings: Excessive action may produce sharp fall in blood pressure and weakness or collapse. Flushing, palpitations may occur.
Administration: Oral, intramuscular, intravenous, intra-arterial.
Preparations: Tablet, 25 mg. Elixir, 25 mg. per 4 cc. Ampule, 10 cc. size, 25 mg. per cc.
Dose: As indicated by need.

TOLBUTAMIDE—Orinase®
New oral insulin substitute.

TOLONIUM—Blutene®
Antimenorrhagic. Green dye.
Actions and Uses: Antiheparin effect which may be useful in treatment and prevention of excessive menstrual flow.
Warnings: If prompt results are not obtained use other measures. Urine turns blue-green. May cause burning on urination.
Administration: Oral.
Preparations: Tablet, 100 mg.
Dose: 200 to 300 mg. daily, before or during menstruation.

TOLOXYN®, see Mephenesin
TOLSERAM®, see Mephenesin
TOLSEROL®, see Mephenesin
TOLU BALSAM
Flavor. Brown plastic solid with pleasant odor and mild taste. Soluble in alcohol.
Actions and Uses: Flavoring agent.
Preparations: Syrup and tincture.
Dose: Syrup, 10 cc. Tincture, 2 cc.

TOLUENE—Toluol
Solvent. Occasionally used as a cleansing agent, but never internally. Highly toxic.

TOLULEXIN®, see Mephenesin

TOLULOX®, see Mephenesin

TOLYSPAZ®, see Mephenesin

TOPITRACIN®, see Bacitracin

TORYN®, see Caramiphen

TOTAQUINE
Antimalarial. A mixture of cinchona alkaloids obtained by partial purification of the cinchona bark.
Actions and Uses: About 75% as effective as quinine in malaria, and if the dose is proportionately raised, has no disadvantages. It was designed for use because it is much cheaper than the purified quinine alkaloid. It has largely been replaced by the more effective recent antimalarial agents.
Preparations: Tablet and capsule.
Dose: 0.6 Gm.

TRAGACANTH
Emulsifier. Used in pharmaceutical preparations and for emulsification.

TRAL®, see Hexocyclium

TRANQUILIZERS
A group of drugs said to affect depression of the higher centers in such a way as to reduce or alleviate tensions and symptoms of anxiety without, at the same time, inducing hypnosis or drowsiness, thereby differing in action from that of the barbiturates and other common sedatives and hypnotics. Many of these drugs also induce a degree of skeletal muscle relaxation. The final results of the present indiscriminate use of these drugs remains to be determined. It is not established, for example, that no addiction liability attends the continued use of these drugs. The value of these agents in the treatment of psychotic patients is reasonably well established but their value in the treatment of the every day run-of-the-mill anxiety symptoms is highly questionable and may even be hazardous in the long run. Acetylcarbromal, Azacyclonal, Benactyzine, Chlorpromazine, Deserpidine, Ectylurea, Hydroxyzine, Mepazine, Meprobamate, Mephenesin, Perphenazine, Phenaglycodol, Proclorperazine, Promazine, Rauwolfia materials, Rescinnamine.

TRASENTINE®, see Adiphenine

TRAVAMIN®, see Plasma Hydrolysate

TRAVERT®, see Invert Sugar

TRIAMCINOLONE—Aristocort®
Anti-inflammatory hormone. Not yet available on the commercial drug market.

TRIASYN B
Vitamin.
Actions and Uses: Capsules or tablets containing a mixture of thiamin (2 mg.), riboflavin (3 mg.) and nicotinamide (20 mg.). Used for combined deficiency disease. Each dose consists of approximately the daily requirements of these vitamins for an adult.

TRIBROMOETHANOL—
Avertin®
Basal anesthetic. White powder with aromatic odor and taste which dissolves in amylene hydrate.
Absorption: Well absorbed from rectum and sigmoid.
Actions and Uses: Originally used for surgical anesthesia and found to be too toxic. More recently used for induction only. Given by enema in the patient's room, it avoids the anxieties which are produced in bringing the patient into the operating room.
Warnings: Not safe as sole agent for surgical anesthesia. Total dose must not exceed 8 cc. for females, 10 cc. for males. Contraindicated in liver disease, severe hypertension, disease of the rectum or colon, advanced pulmonary disease, severe heart disease. Sudden lowering of blood pressure and depression of respiration may occur. In event of overaction, wash out rectum promptly. Store in cool, dark place. Before using, test for decomposition with congo red test solution.
Administration: Rectal.
Preparations: 100 cc. bottle, usually supplied with a small vial of congo red test solution.

Dose: 0.08 cc. to 0.1 cc. per Kg. body weight.
Antidote: Epinephrine.

TRICHLOROETHYLENE—
Trilene®
Anesthetic. Clear colorless liquid with characteristic odor.
Actions and Uses: Highly caustic agent Not frequently used at present.
Warnings: As for all general anesthetics.
Administration: Inhalation.

TRICHLOROACETIC ACID
Caustic. Colorless crystals with characteristic odor. Soluble in water.
Actions and Uses: General anesthetic. used for removal of warts and skin lesions. Also coagulates blood and used as a hemostatic.
Warnings: Not used internally. Apply only to small areas of the skin. Protect other areas with petrolatum. Do not use on skin neoplasms or pigmented moles.
Administration: Topical.
Preparations: Solution.
Dose: Concentration, 50% or milder depending on lesions treated.

TRICOFURON®, see **Furazolidone**

TRICOLOID®, see **Tricyclamol**

TRICYCLAMOL — Elorine®, Tricoloid®
One of the long list of anticholinergic drugs with much the same actions and dangers as atropine, which see.

TRIDIHEXIDE—Pathilon®
One of a large series of anticholinergic agents, which see. Dosage of the order of 25 mg.

TRIDIONE®, see **Trimethadione**

TRIETHANOLAMINE
Emulsifier.
Actions and Uses: Emulsifying agent in the preparation of ointments.

TRIETHANOLAMINE TRINI-TRATE — Metamine®, Nitretamin®
One of the long-acting nitrites. See Nitrites.

TRIETHYLENE MELAMINE—
Melamine, TEM
Anticarcinogenic. Ethylene derivative of nitrogen mustard. See Mechlorethamine. Recommended for treatment of inoperable ovarian carcinoma and other malignancies.

TRIHEXYPHENIDYL—Artane®
Muscle relaxant, anticholinergic. White, odorless solid, soluble in alcohol. The hydrochloride.
Absorption: Well absorbed from the G.I. tract.
Actions and Uses: An atropine-like drug with a well-developed action on smooth muscle as well. It also relieves striated-muscle spasm for reasons which are less well established. This effect which is also found in belladonna derivatives is unpleasant to elicit because of the intense dryness in the mouth and visual disturbances which follow. In the case of the trihexyphenidyl these side effects, while often present, are not usually as intense when muscle relaxation is produced. It finds its greatest use, therefore, in the treatment of the muscle rigidity of Parkinson's Disease.
Warnings: May cause cycloplegia and, in sensitive patients, may induce acute glaucoma. Also may cause mental confusion, nausea, vomiting, agitation.
Administration: Oral.
Preparations: Elixir, 0.5 mg. per cc. Tablets, 2 and 5 mg.
Dose: 1 mg. on first day, 2 mg. on second day, and then 2 mg. increments to a maximum of 6 to 10 mg. daily or less if therapeutic effects are achieved or toxic effects develop.

TRILAFON®, see **Perphenazine**

TRILENE®, see **Trichloroethylene**

TRIMETHADIONE—Tridione®
Anticonvulsant. White granules, camphor-like odor. Soluble in water.
Absorption: Absorbed from G. I. tract.
Actions and Uses: Effective against petit mal type of epilepsy. Sometimes used together with diphenylhydantoin for grand mal epilepsy.

145

Warnings: Blood should be carefully watched for dyscrasias. May also cause gastric irritation, nausea, skin eruptions, light sensitivity and defects in vision.
Administration: Oral.
Preparations: Capsule and tablet.
Dose: 1.0–2.0 Gm. daily in divided doses.

TRIMETON®, see Pheniramine

TRINITROPHENOL—Picric Acid
Antiseptic. Yellow dye. Highly toxic. Little used.

TRIONAMIDE®, see Trisulfapyrimidines

TRIOXYMETHYLENE, see Paraformaldehyde

TRIPAZINE®, see Trisulfapyrimidines

TRIPELENNAMINE — Pyribenzamine®
One of the large series of antihistamine drugs, which see.

TRIPLE BROMIDE, see Bromides

TRISULFAPYRIMIDINES—Methamerdiazine®, Sulfatriazine®, Terfonyl®, Trionamide®, Tripazine®, Tri-sulfameth®, Tri-sulfazine®
Sulfonamide mixture. Equal parts of sulfadiazine, sulfamerazine and sulfamethazine.

TRI-SULFAZINE®, see Trisulfapyrimidines

TRITHEON®, see Aminitrozole

TROMEXAN®, see Ethyl Biscoumacetate

TRONOTHANE®, see Pramoxine
TRI-SULFAMETH®, see Trisulfapyrimidines

TRYPARSAMIDE
Antiluetic and arsenical. Formerly used in treatment of central nervous system syphilis. Largely replaced by penicillin. Highly toxic. See Arsenic.

TRYPSIN, CRYSTALLINE — Parenzyme®, Tryptar®
Purified proteolytic enzyme recommended for local inflammations, especially those of vascular origin. Administered intramuscularly in dosage of from 2-5 mg.

TRYPTAR®, see Trypsin, Crystalline

TUAMINE®, see Tuaminoheptane

TUAMINOHEPTANE—Tuamine®
Adrenergic and nasal decongestant. White powder, the sulfate is soluble in water.
Actions and Uses: Vasoconstrictor and adrenergic drug, with much the same actions as ephedrine.
Warnings: Use with caution in patients with cardiovascular disease.
Administration: Inhalation, topical.
Preparations: Inhaler. Solution, 1 and 2%.
Dose: Depends on indication.

TUBOCURARINE
Muscle relaxant. White to tan powder, soluble in water. Expressed in weight and units.
Actions and Uses: Relaxes skeletal muscle by paralytic action. Used in surgery to complete relaxation of abdominal muscles, in orthopedics in acute poliomyelitis and as a diagnostic agent in myasthenia gravis; in shock therapy to prevent fractures during convulsion.
Warnings: Overdosage may induce loss of diaphragmatic movements and asphyxia. Patient must be watched after its use until normal respiration has fully returned.
Adminstration: Intravenous, intramuscular.
Preparations: Vial, 10 cc. 3 mg. (20 Units) per cc.
Dose: Varies widely with degree of effect desired.
Antidote: Neostigmine.

TURPENTINE OIL
Counterirritant. Colorless liquid, with characteristic odor.
Actions and Uses: Externally as counterirritant. Rectally for pinworms and tympanites.
Warnings: Inflammable. Inhalation of fumes may induce toxic effects. Internal use may cause nephritis.

Administration: Topical, rectal, inhalation.
Preparations: As such.
Dose: Depends upon use. 15–60 cc. in enema for pinworms, constipation, tympanites.

TYLENOL®, see Acetyl-p-aminiphenol

TYROTHRICIN—Soluthricin®
Antibiotic derived from growth of Bacillus brevis. Highly toxic systemically and used only for local application in ointments and solutions.

TYROTHRICIN SOLUTION
Antibiotic. White powder. Insoluble in water.
Actions and Uses: Externally only for infected wounds due to pneumococci, streptococci or staphylococci. Has no important advantages over other antibiotics.
Warnings: Highly toxic intravenously. Ineffective by mouth. Solutions should be refrigerated.
Administration: Topical.
cc. of solution with 0.5 mg. tyrothricin per cc.
Dose: Concentration, 1:2000.

TYVID®, see Isoniazid

TYZINE®, see Tetrahydrozolidine

U

ULTRAN®, see Phenaglycodol

UNDECYLENIC ACID
Fungicide. Yellow liquid, characteristic odor, insoluble in water.
Actions and Uses: Same as zinc undecylenate.

UNDIGIN®, see Digitoxin

UNITENSIN®, see Cryptenamine

UREA—Carbamide
Diuretic. White crystals, soluble in water, characteristic unpleasant taste.
Actions and Uses: In large doses, used as a diuretic, also to dissolve necrotic insufficiency.
Administration: Oral, topical.

Preparations: As such and as solution, 5–50%.
Dose: Oral, 8 Gm. (or more) several times daily.

UREA AND QUININE HYDRO-CHLORIDE, see Quinine and Urea Hydrochloride

URECHOLINE®, see Bethanechol

URETHANE
Sedative and chemotherapeutic. White powder or colorless crystals, soluble in water, saline taste.
Absorption: From G. I. tract.
Actions and Uses: Hypnotic, but mainly used because of characteristic chemotherapeutic action in leukemia.
Warnings: Not dependable as a hypnotic. Not a cure for leukemia.
Administration: Oral, intravenous.
Preparations: Capsule, 0.3 Gm. Ampule, 2 cc. contains 0.3 Gm.
Dose: Oral, 3–5 Gm. daily. Intravenous, 1–3 Gm. daily.

URGININ
Digitalis material. Digitalis glycoside extracted from *Urginea maritima*, Squill, with more rapid action than digitalis leaf or digitoxin but not well absorbed from G.I. tract. See Digitalis.

UROKON®, see Acetrizoate

UROSULFIN®, see Phenazothiadiazole

UROTROPIN®, see Methenamine

V

VALERIAN
An archaic remedy which is probably never used in dosage that produces a pharmacologic effect but, because of its startling taste, is used for placebo.

VALLESTRIL®, see Methallenestril

VALMID®, see Ethinamate

VANILLA
Flavor.

VANILLIN
Flavor.

VANQUIN®, see Pyrvinium

VANZOATE®, see Benzyl Benzoate

VASODILATORS
Adrenolytic drugs, Aminophylline, Aze-petine, Beta-pyridyl carbinol, Betazole, Depropanex®, Hexamethonium, Hista-mine, Methacholine, Nicotinic acid, Ni-trites, Nylidrin, Papaverine, Xanthines.

VASOPRESSIN—Pitressin®
Hormone. As such and as tannate; the former is soluble in water; standardized in U.S.P. Units. Obtained from pituitary extract.
Actions and Uses: Support blood pres-sure, increase activity of bladder and intestine, and in the treatment of diabetes insipidus. The tannate in oil is a depot form for prolonged effects, especially use-ful, in treatment of diabetes insipidus. Has the pressor actions of posterior pituitary extract.
Warnings: Excessive action, especially in patients with heart disease, may be dan-gerous. May cause intestinal cramps, shock-like reaction. Store in cool place and protect from light.
Administration: Intramuscular.
Preparations: Solution, in water (20 U.S.P. Units per cc.) Oil suspension, contains 5 U.S.P. Units per cc. Ampule, contains 1 cc.
Dose: 0.3 to 1.0 cc., repeated as necessary.

VASOXYL®, see Methoxamine

V-CILLIN®, see Phenoxymethyl Penicillin

VERALBA®, see Protoveratrines A and B

VERATRUM PREPARATIONS
Cryptenamine, Protoveratrines A and B.

VERATRUM VIRIDE—
Hellebore
Hypotensive. Brown powder, bitter taste; standardized in Craw Units.
Actions and Uses: At this time there is a revival of an old practice to use this drug for its hypotensive actions. In the main, there is little evidence to support such use for the drug, and it may well be, that this use comes from the fact that there is so little that can be done for most patients with hypertension, that al-most anything will be tried, especially, as in this case, with a drug which has no particular dangers.
Warnings: Often causes G. I. distress. Often given together with a barbiturate.
Administration: Oral.
Preparations: There are many, usually tablets. Often mixtures with hypnotics and sedatives, from which it is likely that the mixtures obtain most of their effects.
Dose: 10 or more Craw Units, several times daily.

VERMIZINE®, see Piperazine

VERONAL®, see Barbital

VERSENE®, see Edathamil

VIADRIL®, see Hydroxydione

VIBAZINE®, see Buclizine

VIBURNUM
Placebo.
Actions and Uses: There are at least two species of this material, and many preparations, recommended as a tonic, for uterine cramps, antispasmodic, abor-tion, etc. These preparations all have an intensely bitter taste, and it seems likely, since there is no evidence that they have any pharmacologic action, that all their effects derive from the psychologic effects of the bitter taste. Valerian, also an old remedy for the same conditions, probably has the same kind of action.

VINACTANE®, see Viomycin

VINBARBITAL—Delvinal®
One of the intermediate acting barbitu-rates, which see.

VINETHENE®, see Vinyl Ether

VINISIL®, see Polyvidone

VINYL ETHER—Vinethene®,
Divinyl Ether
Anesthetic. Clear liquid with characteris-tic odor.

Actions and Uses: Used for general anesthesia of short duration, such as dental procedures. Also used as an induction anesthetic.

Warnings: Explosive. Over use may cause liver damage. Difficult to manage because of rapidity of action. Refrigerate.

Administration: Inhalation (usually drop).

Preparations: Solution.

Dose: Determined by anesthetist and situation. About 5 cc. usually.

VIOCIN®, see Viomycin

VIOFORM®, see Iodochlorhydroxyquin

VIOMYCIN—Vinactane®, Viocin®
Antibiotic. Isolated from a fungus. The sulfate, soluble in water.

Actions and Uses: Exerts an action against the tubercle bacillus and used, therefore, in cases of tuberculosis resistant to streptomycin, isoniazid, or para-aminosalicylic acid treatment, or in combination with them.

Warnings: A new drug, relatively untested.

Administration: Intramuscular.

Preparations: Vials containing 1 Gm.

Dose: 2 Gm. every third day.

VIOSTEROL, see Synthetic Oleovitamin D

VISAMMIN — Amnivin®, Khelisem®, Khellin
Vasodilator. Extract of Egyptian plant *Amni visnaga* said to relieve pain of coronary spasm by vasodilatation. Careful examination in well-controlled studies, however, fails to reveal an effect beyond that of placebo.

VITAMIN A, see Oleovitamin A

VITAMIN B₁, see Thiamin

VITAMIN B₂, see Riboflavin

VITAMIN B₆, see Pyridoxine

VITAMIN B₁₂ — Cyanocobalamin, Bevidox®, Rametin®, Redisol®
Nutritional and hematinic. Red crystals or powder. Soluble in water.

Absorption: From G. I. tract.

Actions and Uses: Apparently identical with antianemic factor of liver. Used in managemnt of pernicious anemia and other macrocytic anemias, sprue, megaloblastic anemia of infants. Useful especially in patients who cannot tolerate liver.

Warnings: Refrigerate. Protect from light.

Preparations: Sterile aqueous solution, 10 cc. vial containing 15 µg. per cc.

Dose: Variable as indicated.

VITAMIN B COMPLEX—Brewer's Yeast
Nutritional.

Actions and Uses: A mixture of thiamin, riboflavin, niacinamide, pantothenic acid, pyridoxine and other yeast extractives. Used to treat deficiencies.

Administration: Oral, parenteral.

Preparations: Flavored syrups, powders, capsules, drops, tablets, etc.

VITAMIN C, see Ascorbic Acid

VITAMIN D—Synthetic Oleovitamin D, Calciferol, Viosterol, Drisdol® There are a large number of phenanthrene derivatives which exert the actions on calcium metabolism and bone growth which are characteristic of Vitamin D. These may be derived from natural sources, chiefly from fish-liver oils, or like Calciferol are made synthetically. At present the synthetic materials are probably used more than the natural Vitamin D. There are no important differences in therapeutic effects and the lack of taste of the former is a practical advantage. Synthetic Oleovitamin D, the official preparation, must be labelled to indicate whether it contains calciferol or its vitamin D acitivity derives from other forms of Vitamin D. See Synthetic Oleovitamin D.

VITAMIN E—Mixed Tocopherols
Although this vitamin is essential for reproduction in the rat, there is no evidence that this applies to the human or that the tocopherols are of any value in diseases of humans.

VITAMIN G, see Riboflavin

VITAMIN K, see Menadione

VITAMIN K$_1$, see Phytonadione

VITAMIN PREPARATIONS

There is such a large number of vitamin preparations, pure, mixtures, various strengths and combinations, combinations with other nonvitamin materials, official and nonofficial preparations, commercial preparations with different names and different claims, that no attempt can be made to list even a small percentage of them all.

There is no evidence that vitamins help any situation other than those in which they are specifically needed. The only indications, therefore, are as a prophylactic effect on the patient, and in actual vitamin deficiency conditions in which they may cure the disease. Vitamins have no tonic or stimulatory effect in diseases not associated with nutritional deficiency. Vitamin deficiency may result from poor diet, through poverty, ignorance, special diets for reducing, etc. and disease which prevents the absorption of vitamins.

Large amounts of vitamins are taken by a large proportion of our population at great expense with little value. In some, the cost is justified by prophylactic action of vitamins, and those who take them for this reason are perhaps getting some of their money's worth. In a few instances, they are used for bona fide vitamin deficiencies, but for the most part, this large sum of money is expended by patients for a remedy which can exert only a placebo action, this latter action having been established because of the large amount of loose talk about the general nonspecific values of vitamins.

The following is a list of some of the materials which have been designated as vitamins. Many of them are not in common use either because clinical deficiency of this vitamin never or very rarely occurs in man or because the vitamin is of no value when the deficiency occurs.

Adenylic acid, Ascorbic acid, Avidin, Biotin, Calciferol, Carotene, Choline, Dihydrotachysterol, Factor T, Folic acid, Inositol, Nicotinamide (Niacinamide), Nicotinic acid, Oleovitamin D, Paraaminobenzoic acid, Pantothenic acid, Phytonadione, Provitamin A, Pyridoxine, Riboflavin, Vitamin A, Vitamin B complex, Vitamin B$_{12}$, Vitamin D, Vitamin E, Vitamin K, Vitamin P.

VITAMIN SUPPLEMENTS

Actions and Uses: Usually a mixture containing all or a stated fraction of the established daily adult requirements of the identified vitamins. Used as supplements to the diet.

VONEDRINE®, see Phenylpropylmethylamine

W

WARFARIN—Coumadin®, Prothromadin®

Anticoagulant. Originally used as a rodenticide because of this property but more recently introduced into medicine. May be administered intravenously, thereby acting more rapidly than the usual coumarin derivatives. Also relatively rap-long-lasting; a single oral dose may produce a depression of prothrombin lasting about 3 days. Doses should be spaced accordingly. Intravenous dose of the order of 60 to 75 mg.; oral dosage about 25 to 50 mg. every 3 or 4 days. Prothrombin levels must be determined frequently for safe use.

WASHING SODA, see Sodium Carbonate

WATER FOR INJECTION

Actions and Uses: Although ordinary idly absorbed from G.I. tract. Effects are distilled water may be used for oral preparations of pharmaceuticals, this is often not pure enough for parenteral preparations. When large amounts are injected intravenously, febrile reactions may result from distilled water alone. Febrile reactions from water are due to unidentified materials called pyrogens. Pyrogen-free water is obtained by distillation under special conditions and only this form should be used for intravenous injection.

WAX
Pharmaceutic. Used in ointments, plasters, etc. to give body to the preparation.

WHISKEY—Spiritus Frumenti
Sedative. See alcohol.

WHITE PETROLATUM, see Petrolatum

WHITE PINE
Expectorant.
Actions and Uses: Used mainly in proprietary cough mixtures. Of doubtful value.

WHITE PRECIPITATE, see Ammoniated Mercury

WHITFIELD'S OINTMENT, see Benzoic and Salicylic Acid Ointment

WILD CHERRY SYRUP—
Cherry, Wild
Flavor: Common flavor for cough syrup.

WINTERGREEN OIL, see Methyl Salicylate

WOOL FAT—Lanolin
Base. Fat-like substance which mixes well with water.
Actions and Uses: Used as base for skin preparations, sometimes as such, and often in ointments and other skin preparations. One of its special virtues is its ability to mix with water. Has no special medicinal or curative values.
Preparations: Anhydrous (dry). Hydrous (25-30% water).

WORMSEED OIL, see Chenopodium Oil

WYAMINE®, see Mephentermine

WYDASE®, see Hyaluronidase

X

XANTHINES
Drugs of vegetable origin, commonly found in popular drinks, all of which are closely related to caffeine, all of which are eliminated in the urine in the form of uric acid, and all of which have certain actions in common: (1) central stimulation (excitement, wakefulness, respiratory stimulation), (2) diuresis, (3) vasodilation.
Central stimulation is the quality that makes it attractive in drinks, such as coffee, tea, cocoa. The caffeine in the first two and the theobromine in the third, provide this effect. Caffeine is used for similar reason in medicine.
Diuretic actions without too much central action are well developed in theophylline, and this drug is used for that reason.
Vasodilator action is presumed to be exerted on the coronary vessels, and for that reason, aminophylline has long been used in disease of the coronary arteries. Such an action, while shown to be present under experimental conditions, has not been demonstrated in the presence of arteriosclerosis of the coronary arteries, and the use of aminophylline for this condition is falling into disuse.
Caffeine, Choline theophyllinate, Hyphilline, Theobromine, Theobromine calcium salicylate, Theobromine sodium acetate, Theobromine sodium salicylate. Theophylline compounds are Aminophylline, Theophylline sodium acetate, Theophylline methyl-glucamine, Theophylline-sodium glycinate.

XANTHOTOXIN, see Methoxsalen

XEROFORM®, see Bismuth Tribromophenate

XYLENE—Xylol
Solvent. Used in the laboratory. Not used internally. Highly toxic.

XYLOCAINE®, see Lidocaine

Y

YATREN®, see Chiniofon
YEAST, BREWER'S
Actions and Uses: A crude, but otherwise adequate and complete source of

151

Z.P.O.

Vitamin B complex. See Vitamin B Complex.

YERBA SANTA, see Eriodictyon

YODOXIN®, see Diiodohydroxyquinoline

Z

ZEPHIRAN®, see Benzalkonium

ZINADON®, see Isoniazid

ZINAX BURN DRESSING®, see Zinc Acetate

ZINC ACETATE
Dressing. White crystalline solid, soluble in water and alcohol.
Actions and Uses: Used in the preparation of a burn dressing which is impregnated in gauze.

ZINC IODIDE AND IODINE GLYCERITE, see Iodine

ZINC OINTMENT, see Zinc Oxide

ZINC OXIDE
Astringent and antiseptic. White powder, insoluble in water.
Actions and Uses: Used in skin conditions and in dusting powders as a protective.
Administration: Topical.
Preparations: Zinc gelatin, zinc oxide pastes (Lassar's), Unna's boot (hard and soft), zinc oxide paste with salicylic acid, ointment, zinc oxide and castor oil, zinc oxide and Juniper tar.
Dose: Concentration, 20–25%.

ZINC PASTE, see Zinc Oxide

ZINC PEROXIDE—Z.P.O
Oxidant and antiseptic. White powder, insoluble in water.
Actions and Uses: Liberates oxygen slowly. Used as antiseptic agent for putrid infections.
Warnings: Unstable. Applications usually are active not more than 24 hours. Do

not use moist powders. Seal containers. Store in dry place.
Administration: Topical.
Preparations: Cream and powder.
Dose: Concentration, 40%.

ZINC STEARATE
Skin protective. White powder.
Actions and Uses: Astringent. Emetic. Used mainly as a skin protective.
Warnings: Dust is irritant to lungs and may cause serious reactions.

ZINC SULFATE
Astringent. Colorless crystals, soluble in water.
Actions and Uses: Used mainly in eye washes for astringent and antiseptic action. Also used occasionally as an emetic.
Warnings: May irritate eye if used in concentrations above 0.2%.
Administration: Topical, oral (if retained when used as emetic, wash stomach).
Preparations: Eye wash and drops.
Dose: Eye, concentration of 0.2%. Emetic, 1 Gm.

ZINC UNDECYLENATE
Fungicide. White powder, insoluble in water.
Actions and Uses: Prophylaxis and treatment of dermatophytosis and other skin diseases caused by fungi.
Warnings: Store in dry place.
Administration: Topical.
Preparations: Powder and ointment. Also usually contains undecylenic acid which has much the same action on fungi.
Dose: Concentration, 20%.

ZOXAZOLAMINE—Flexin®
Skeletal muscle relaxant.
Actions and Uses: "Lissive", said to relieve skeletal muscle spasm and, in contrast to other drugs, without interfering with normal muscle function.
Warnings: A new drug, yet to be clearly evaluated.
Administration: Oral.
Preparations: 250 mg. tablets (yellow).
Dose: 250–500 mg. 3 to 4 times a day.

Z.P.O., see Zinc Peroxide.